The Fat Burning Diet

The Fat Burning Diet

Accessing Unlimited Energy
For a Lifetime

Jay Robb

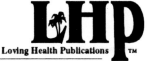

"Publications that share the wealth of health"

Box 711533 • Santee, California 92072

Robb, Jay
The Fat Burning Diet
Accessing Unlimited Energy for a Lifetime / Jay Robb

ISBN 0-9620608-1-X
1. Reducing diets. 2. Nutrition. 3. Diet—popular works.

Manufactured in the United States of America

Loving Health Publications
Box 711533
Santee, CA 92072-1533

Dedicated to my best friend Bruce Heflebower
From the moment we first met at Jay's Gym you have been an
inspiration and a guiding light in my fitness journey. From Baja to
our many ha-has, you will always be my brother; my *Fat Burner
Brother.*

A Special Thank You to my dear wife **Rosemary Castagna Robb**,
my loving son **Angelo Joseph Robb**, our English Springer
"Jacquemo" and our gray cheek parrot **"Geppetto,"** for tolerat-
ing my absence as a husband and father during my seemingly endless years of work-work-work while I developed *Jay Robb Enterprises* and researched, and completed this book. You are all a
contributing factor for my desire to accomplish more and do greater
things...

And thank you: Joyce "Mama" Robb for your unconditional love,
endless support and encouragement; Robert Harris for your editing skills, legal advice, inspiring humor and long distance friend-
ship; C. J. Hunt for your editing skills and promotional help; and
to my worldwide friends and supporters, *God Bless you all...*

Acknowledgements:

Special thanks to the following individuals. In a world that is addicted to carbohydrates and petrified of fats, these doctors and researchers are true fat burning pioneers.

Dr. Gregory Ellis, Ph.D.

Thank you for your endless research into the field of fat burning and carbohydrate restricted diets.

Dr. Robert Atkins, MD.

Thank you for your wonderful books and persistence on teaching the truth about diet and the problems of consuming too many carbohydrates.

Dr. Cass Igram

Thank you for your inspiring book, *Eat Right or Die Young*, and for teaching the world that the consumption of excess sugars and starches is the real cause of many of our degenerative diseases.

Dr. Barry Sears

Thank you for your work with endurance athletes and your many articles that have inspired me to continue teaching the "real" fat burning secrets.

Dr. Phillip Maffetone

Thank you for your specialized work with endurance athletes and for telling the world to eat less carbohydrate and more "natural" fat to enhance the fat burning process.

Author's Note

This book is offered to you on the following principles:
1. I don't claim to know it all.
2. I'm always learning.
3. I have a very important message to share with you at this present moment.

The author does not claim to be a doctor or healer of any sort. This book is intended for educational purposes only and should not be used as a guide for diagnosis and treatment of any disease. If you have any health problems, it is advisable to seek the advice of a health care professional of your choice.

Note: Unless otherwise stated, all quotes in this book are the author's.

Contents

Chapters:

Page

Introduction.. 9
1. Why Burn Fat?... 13
2. The Carbohydrate Myth...................................... 15
3. Hypoglycemia, Diabetes and Insulin.................. 20
4. Breaking the Carbohydrate Addiction................ 25
5. Fat Burning Principles.. 29
6. The Fat Burning Diet.. 34
7. Fat Burning Menu Ideas..................................... 44
8. Creating Your Own Meals.................................. 65
9. Cholesterol Is Your Friend, Not Your Enemy.... 73
10. Food Combining... 77
11. Your Support System.. 81
12. Candida, Lactobacteria and Colon Health........ 83
13. Fat Burning for the Whole Family.................... 88
14. Exercises That Burn Fat.................................... 91
15. Fat Burning For Bodybuilders and Athletes...... 95
16. Flaxing Your Muscles....................................... 98
17. Delicious Fat Burning Recipes....................... 101
18. Mini-Cleanses for Maximum Health.............. 120
19. Nutritional Supplements................................. 121
20. Fat Burning Questions and Answers............... 124
21. In Summary.. 129
22. In Closing. A Personal Testimonial................ 132
References... 135

Introduction

A man strolls into his favorite drinking establishment, settles onto a vacant bar stool and orders an ice cold brew. Within moments, he is approached by an attractive young woman wearing a very revealing outfit. Portraying sensual body language, this breathtaking beauty leans forward and whispers into the man's ear, "For $50 I'll do anything you desire, but you must tell me your desire in three words or less."

Having just stormed out of the house, after a disagreement with his wife, the man's ears perked up a bit. But control and self discipline outweighed the tempting request, so the man remained quiet and stared straight ahead at his beer.

Again the woman leans forward and softly whispers into his ear, "For $50 I'll do anything you desire, but you must tell me your desire in three words or less." The man's ears began twitching as the soft words made his body tingle. But, once again, his masterful control stopped him from moving even an inch.

Sensing the man's resistance to be weakening, the tempting female goddess again leans forward, this time purposely brushing her soft upper body against his shoulder as she whispered her provocative offer into his ear, "For $50 I'll do anything you desire, but you must tell me your desire in three words or less."

That was it! The man's resistance crumbled as he realized this offer was simply too good to let pass by. Quickly rising from his bar stool, the man slipped a $50 bill into her awaiting palm, leaned forward and whispered softly into her ear, "Paint my house."

Everyday of our life we make choices. As the story above illustrates, we have many options in all situations. All too often our mind goes into tunnel vision and only sees the obvious, thus we overlook other possibilities that could have "better served our desires." This book is about being open to other possibilities and thinking for ourselves instead of always going along with the crowd.

Diet and health are two of the most controversial and highly debated subjects in America (next to religion and politics). But amidst all the controversy, the simple unchangeable truth exists. *The Fat Burning Diet* is my way of offering this simple dietary truth to you.

Requiring over 16 years to develop and perfect, *The Fat Burning Diet* outperforms any other diet ever conceived. Offering unlimited energy, delicious and satisfying meals, optimum nutrition, mental clarity, blood sugar stabilization, ample protein and plenty of flexibility, *The Fat Burning Diet* is an ideal way of eating that unleashes the energy dynamo that resides within you.

And don't even, for one tiny moment, think that this diet is only a weight loss plan. *The Fat Burning Diet* is for everyone (from athletes to executives to homemakers) who desires to tap into their ultimate fuel source, which is fat, thus supplying their body with optimum energy for life. When you burn fat for fuel, there are no "ups" and "downs" as are so common with carbohydrate-based diets. Once you apply the fat burning principles to your life, the sky is the limit! If excess bodyfat and/or low energy has stopped you from succeeding in the past, then get ready to "sizzle" your way to the top! That's my promise to you...

Naturally,

Jay Robb
Your Fat Burning Friend

"A Quitter Never Wins And A Winner Never Quits."
— Napolean Hill

Chapter 1

Why Burn Fat?

What if you had the opportunity to experience one day of your life where you had a steady supply of energy with no fatigue, no hunger, no cravings, and absolutely no mood swings. Your day would begin by leaping out of bed, alert, full of energy and ready to dance through the day. Now imagine your steady supply of uninterrupted energy was coming directly from your own bodyfat stores. Sound wonderful? It is and I invite everyone to experience this natural phenomenon: "fat burning."

How has such a simple physical process such as burning one's own bodyfat become so difficult? The answer is twofold:

1. Americans consume excess quantities of carbohydrate foods.
2. Americans don't move their bodies as much as they could or should.

Once a person understands what is needed to burn bodyfat for fuel, one's whole life changes. Many Americans don't pursue their dreams or reach their goals because they lack vital energy. Millions of Americans are slaves to their diet and are unknowingly addicted to many foods that are high in carbohydrate (for example: soda pop, bread, potatoes, chocolate, sugar, juice, cookies, cakes, fruit, pies, candy bars, pizza crust, pasta, ice cream, etc.).

Four reasons to burn fat as energy:

1. Fat is a long burning energy source that doesn't let you down (no mood swings, no energy slumps).
2. Fat burning keeps a person's fat stores in constant check.
3. Fat burning allows you to exercise for long periods without experiencing fatigue or "hitting the wall." A long distance runner possessing a mere 8% bodyfat will have approximately 10-15 times as much energy stored as fat than as carbohydrate. Stop carbohydrate loading and BURN FAT!
4. Fat is the body's fuel of choice, not carbohydrate, as many erroneously believe. Give your body what it prefers!
5. Fat is down right fun to burn, and the pleasure of seeing your bodyfat levels plunge is truly a delight.

Very few individuals know the secrets to burning fat. Many try to exercise fat away by performing marathon workouts, while others try to starve themselves in hopes of losing fat forever. There is a better way to tap into your own bodyfat reserves and this book reveals those secrets to you. Let's now take a look at carbohydrates, which for countless years have been a fat burning obstacle to millions of Americans...

Chapter 2

The Carbohydrate Myth

"Many people believe that carbohydrate is the primary fuel for the body. However, this belief is not true. The primary fuel for the body is fat." — Gregory S. Ellis, Ph.D.

How many times have you heard or read that one should be eating plenty of complex carbohydrates while simultaneously cutting out almost all dietary fats? And the alleged outcome of this dietary adjustment is a body filled with energy and trimmed of excess fat. Sound logical? At first glimpse it does, but then Custer too thought he was doing the logical thing at Little Big Horn.

What are carbohydrates? Many of us aren't quite aware that a large percentage of the food we consume is really some form of carbohydrate. From pasta to popcorn, and pickles to pretzels, carbohydrates are everywhere.

The following is a partial list of common carbohydrate foods that are consumed daily by the average American:

bread	syrup	candy bars
pasta	pancakes	cereal
potatoes	waffles	all grains
French fries	yams	tortillas
fruit	squash	beans
fruit juice	potato chips	vegetables
sugar	doughnuts	ice cream
soda pop	candy	

Many other carbohydrate foods also appear in our diet as "hidden sugars" and may be found on labels in the following forms:

fructose	maltodextrin	raw sugar
glucose	glucose polymers	turbinado sugar
dextrose	barley malt	dried cane juice
maltose	date sugar	
lactose	honey	

Carbohydrates are a food source that, once ingested, must be broken down to glucose (a simple sugar) by a special enzymatic process. Once carbohydrate is converted to glucose, the bloodstream becomes the vehicle to transport the simple sugar throughout the body, in hopes of being burned as fuel. If only a small amount of carbohydrate is ingested, then only a small amount of glucose is created and dispensed into the bloodstream. For general energy needs, this small amount of carbohydrate is easily burned and no excess glucose remains in the bloodstream.

But what happens if you were to consume a sizable amount of carbohydrate, such as a plate of pasta; or two baked potatoes; or a bowl of cereal, one banana and 6 ounces of skim milk? Excess glucose is then formed from the large quantity of carbohydrate and unless you are getting ready to dance for two hours, go for a 2-3 mile run, or take a very, very long walk, your bloodstream is going to be flooded with glucose that simply has nowhere to go!

As your blood sugar levels rise, the body signals the pancreas to control the amount of glucose in the bloodstream because, as any diabetic knows, excess glucose in the bloodstream can be dangerous if allowed to remain too high for too long.

After receiving the excess glucose panic signal, the pancreas secretes a powerful hormone called INSULIN, which steps in to: a) make glucose available to the cells for energy, b) convert glucose into glycogen (starch stored in the liver and in the muscles), or c) convert glucose into triglycerides, which is a fancy word for "pre-bodyfat." If a person regularly eats a high carbohydrate diet, chances are their muscles are continually loaded with glycogen. Once muscle glycogen is replenished, the only alternative your body has is to convert all excess glucose into BODYFAT! And the fat your body creates will often be stored in the areas of your body that you least desire.

All Fat Burning Comes To A Screeching Halt!

Once the body generates a blood sugar-stabilizing dose of insulin from the pancreas, ALL FAT BURNING COMES TO AN IMMEDIATE HALT! Why? Because excess glucose in the bloodstream is very dangerous and can lead to cellular dehydration due to osmotic diuresis of the kidneys which causes electrolyte and fluid depletion. Hence, the controlling, anti-fat burning hormone that the body produces is INSULIN, which has the power to keep you from using fat as fuel for quite some time.

Unfortunately, once your bloodstream is cleared of excess glucose by the action of insulin, the body is suddenly robbed of its fuel source. The presence of insulin causes blood sugar levels to return to normal, or sometimes dips them below normal, and this means low or no energy. All fat burning is shut down by the action of insulin so the body has no choice but to seek more "sugar" to burn. Suddenly hunger strikes, usually in the form carbohydrate (sugar) cravings. What will you do? Order a pizza or reach for a candy bar? And once you indulge, the blood sugar, fat storing process is started all over again.

The above process could be equated to someone siphoning all the gas from your automobile and placing it in a storage tank. There is no problem with removing the fuel from your vehicle until you jump in your car to drive across town. What's the problem? You have plenty of gas , but it's in storage and you do not have immediate access to it. What will you do? (call a tow truck and order a pizza!).

The key to fat metabolism (fat burning) is to tightly regulate the amount of carbohydrate consumed so that it precisely correlates with your immediate energy needs. Is it becoming obvious why your present dietary patterns sometimes make you feel like a YO-YO, with NO-NO, GO-GO! Let's face it, once insulin works its magic on excess glucose, you may then experience any one or all of the following:

- Hunger
- Food Cravings
- Sugar Cravings
- Dizziness
- Low Energy
- Mental confusion

- Despair
- Depression
- Anxiety
- Frustration
- Anger
- Weakness

A carbohydrate burner (different from a fat burner) needs to burn glucose as fuel, and this especially includes the brain. The "sugar burner" is basically addicted to carbohydrates and must rely almost exclusively on glucose for all energy needs, unless he or she is performing one or more hours of a cardiovascular exercise per day (more on exercise addiction later). When blood sugar levels are low, the brain of a carbohydrate-dependent individual can become starved for fuel.

"Also interesting and unfortunate for the "sugar burner" is that high levels of insulin in the bloodstream completely shut off all fat mobilizing activities, thus dietary fat gets stored right along with the fat (triglycerides) your liver produced from your last high carbohydrate meal."

Without glucose to power the brain, the reaction may be confusion, depression, despair, fear and anxiety. If you are regularly consuming ample quantities of carbohydrate replete foods, this is what takes place in your body each and every day! Imagine how our children must feel after consuming candy, sodas, ice cream, cookies and junk food each day!

Gas, or flatulence, is another common problem that often plagues a person who consumes high levels of carbohydrates. Ask anyone that is eating a high carbohydrate diet if they ever experience gas or bloating and they are likely to say, "All the time. I'm miserable!" Gas was always a problem for me until I cut out the excess carbohydrates in my diet. It's as simple as that!

Also interesting and unfortunate for the "sugar burner" is that high levels of insulin in the bloodstream completely shut off all fat burning activities, thus dietary fat gets stored right along with the fat (triglycerides) your liver produced from your last high carbohydrate meal.[1] This sounds like a lose-lose situation at first, but once you learn my secrets to burning fat for fuel you will suddenly realize that your fat stores are only a savings account that you can tap into anytime you please.

Most people have no clue as to the severity of their carbohydrate addiction. If you doubt that you could be addicted to carbohydrates, then take the fat burning challenge! Try functioning for one day without drinking or ingesting anything (except water) between breakfast and your evening meal. If your breakfast is a typical American high carbohydrate feast, then you will probably lose your "cool" by 10:00 am., because a carbohydrate meal can let you "down" in approximately 1-2 hours.

"Burning fat is as refreshing as a *cool breeze through a camel's knees.*"

For the "fat burner", life is completely different. Burning fat is as refreshing as a "cool breeze through a camel's knees." Fat-derived energy flows steadily into the bloodstream to fuel the cells and muscles of the body as needed. No ups and no downs, just continual energy all day long. Sound good? It's Grrreat! A true gift from God! But before I let you in on all the secrets to burning fat, let's take a closer look at some of the more serious problems that are associated with a diet that is too rich in carbohydrates...

Chapter 3

Hypoglycemia, Diabetes and Insulin

I began my fat burning learning journey (say that 3 times real fast) in 1978 after being diagnosed as having severe hypoglycemia (low blood sugar). My Preventative Medical Physician advised me to avoid refined carbohydrates, all sugar, white bread and white flour and to also supplement my diet with specific vitamins and minerals. There was only one major problem. As a hard training bodybuilder, I was already doing exactly as my doctor advised and yet my blood sugar levels were still doing the "low yo-yo!"

Crying before a meal was very common to me in 1978, as was feeling depressed, spaced out and full of anxiety. Panic attacks were also a daily affair which caused me to feel scared, weak and physically exhausted. At times I truly feared I was losing my mind!

I can vividly recall collapsing after one of my workouts and the horror that engulfed my cerebral sensors. It was on one of my usual training days when I suddenly began to experience weakness and fatigue like never before. After failing to complete the third repetition on the inclined bench press (with a weight I could have normally completed 12 or more reps), I suddenly lost all my strength as if someone pulled my plug. Repetition three went half way up and then straight back down on my chest and there it stayed! Two fellow "iron pumpers" pulled the crushing weight from my chest and I sat there numb and unable to move.

My mind was racing and the room began to spin. My energy level was non-existent but I somehow managed to grab my training gear, stagger through the door, get in my car and drive home. Feeling dazed, I stumbled into my apartment, headed for the bedroom and literally collapsed. The room was spinning as fear invaded my every thought. Seconds became hours and minutes seemed like days. This moment of my life was worse than all my nightmares combined. This nightmare was real and I couldn't get it to stop!

Later I was to learn that the above experience was a severe blood sugar plunge which caused a physical collapse and extreme mental confusion. It was the horror of that day which inspired me to endlessly search until I discovered the "absolute" truth about my condition (hypoglycemia). And I was not looking to just control this disorder. I wanted to know exactly how to eliminate it for life! My search has not been in vain, for out of my persistence *The Fat Burning Diet* was born!

What Is Hypoglycemia?

Hypoglycemia is an abnormally low level of glucose in the bloodstream, often caused by the consumption of excess carbohydrates, or in certain cases by tumors of the pancreas causing an overproduction of insulin, or by disorders of the liver interfering with the storage and release of glucose.[2]

Low blood sugar actually has a variety of "root" causes, but the utmost reason for blood sugar disorders is the excess consumption of carbohydrates! Food allergies or intolerances can also contribute to dips in blood sugar levels, even if the offending food is not carbohydrate based. In a clinical test, one patient was found to be so sensitive (allergic) to milk that within two hours after consuming a portion of cream cheese (which is only 2% carbohydrate), his blood sugar levels dipped to an extremely low point.[3] Now imagine the double trouble of eating a concentrated carbohydrate food such as wheat and also being allergic to it. That combination could sail you above the clouds and then plunge you to the greatest depths!

While my blood sugar problems in 1978 were quite severe, millions of Americans are presently experiencing mild hypoglycemic symptoms daily and they aren't aware that a problem exists. In fact, when most Americans unknowingly face the "blood sugar blues" they generally reach for: coffee (a stimulant that raises blood sugar levels from the effect of the drug, caffeine); soda pop that often contains sugar and caffeine; tea (a mild blood sugar elevator); a doughnut; gum; candy or any sweet treat that will cause a quick rise in blood sugar levels. Once the coffee or snack is consumed, blood sugar levels increase and the person *feels better* until the next *dip* comes along. This is how a great number of people deal with a disorder they do not understand. Many people believe they keep running out of energy, so they eat sugar or something sweet. And, unless they are very physically active, the carbohydrates in that treat will be rapidly converted to BODYFAT!

Uncontrollable hunger, food cravings, moodiness, anger, rage, crying spells, frustration, fears, lack of energy, apathy, exhaustion, anxiety and mental confusion are a few of the most common low blood sugar symptoms. And hypoglycemia is only the beginning of the problem because in reality, low blood sugar episodes are merely the forerunner to Type II diabetes.[4]

It should now be quite obvious to you that once carbohydrates take over and become a major part of your diet, then look out! Unless you plan on taking a 2-3 mile run after each high carbohydrate meal, there could be blood sugar problems! To prevent and avoid blood sugar trouble, the simple solution is to limit the amount and type of carbohydrates that you consume, thus avoiding all the ups and downs, and I mean UPS and DOWNS! When insulin is only secreted in small amounts, which is what happens on *The Fat Burning Diet,* then there is nearly a zero chance of developing excess bodyfat, hypoglycemia or Type II diabetes (Type I diabetes, or juvenile diabetes is caused by a genetic defect or damage to the pancreas which causes the body to stop producing insulin).

Modern supplements, such as chromium Picolinate, are now available and have been clinically proven to be of benefit to hypoglycemics and early stage Type II hyperglycemics, by restoring some of insulin's efficiency.[5] Chromium is a vital trace mineral that is responsible for insulin's "Glucose Tolerance Factor" (GTF), meaning it is the factor in insulin which acts readily on glucose, thus making it available for energy, reception, mobilization or storage.

While I find chromium Picolinate (elemental chromium bonded with picolinic acid) to be a valuable supplement for restoring usable chromium to individuals who are deficient, (and many recent studies have determined that most individuals are deficient in the essential trace mineral chromium), the use of chromium Picolinate for blood sugar disorders is equated to placing a bandage on a shaving cut which is caused from using a faulty blade. If you shave every day you get cut every day. The bandage (chromium) helps, but it does not remove the underlying cause. Only by removing the faulty blade (a high carbohydrate diet) and replacing it with a new blade (*The Fat Burning Diet*) will you correct the "real" problem. Once the diet is corrected, then in my opinion, chromium Picolinate has a much greater potential for permanently restoring the efficiency of insulin.

Having experienced the perils and actual horror of hypoglycemia, I have compassion for the millions of Americans who experience blood sugar fluctuations on a regular basis. By developing and utilizing *The Fat Burning Diet* principles, I have assured that my blood sugar disorder is now in the past! It's history, it's over, adios, bye-bye, and buenos noches! Burning fat for fuel has changed my life and I now have the energy and inner drive to share this incredible diet plan with the world.

I must make a confession. I made a bargain with the *Universe*. "Lead me to the lifestyle and diet that will end this 'blood sugar roller coaster ride' and I'll spread the news across the land," was my prayer. This book is my end of the bargain and more. Not only was I shown the way out of the depths of hypoglycemia, but I was given an extra bonus of discovering the secrets to burning fat for energy. I truly received more than I asked for and now I'm sharing these secrets with you so that you may do the same. Experience this incredible diet yourself and then please tell a friend.

If you are experiencing hypoglycemia or hyperglycemia (both of which are detected by taking a six hour glucose tolerance test), then please share this book with your doctor and let him/her know that you desire to utilize fat (not carbohydrate) for your energy needs. Your physician should be more than happy to help you overcome your carbohydrate addiction so that you may become a fat burning fireball who is ready to tackle the world!

Chapter 4

Breaking The Carbohydrate Addiction

Breaking any addiction can be very difficult or very easy, and the difference lies entirely in one's mind. Think *difficult thoughts* and sure enough the task is often complicated, frustrating and challenging. Think *easy thoughts* and then it's "smooth sailing."

A woman once asked the famous self-help psychologist Dr. Wayne Dyer, "What obstacles are in the way of my attaining true happiness?" And Dr. Dyer replied, "Only the belief that you must have obstacles. " Nothing else was blocking her path.

"Choose positive thoughts and you will see positive changes."

The first step to breaking a carbohydrate addiction is in thought. Choose positive thoughts and you will see positive changes. If you truly desire to change the quality of your life by tossing the carbohydrate "monkey" off your back, then simply change the way you think.

It is of utmost importance that you admit to yourself and others that you are carbohydrate dependent. It is secondly important that you understand that FAT is your primary source of fuel, not carbohydrate. You must stop viewing carbohydrate as your energy source! FAT IS YOUR PREDOMINANT SOURCE OF ENERGY! And please, this is not a war against carbohydrates. "Carbs" are not bad guys, they just are not our #1 source of sustained energy. Finally, you must make a serious commitment to become a Fat Burner for life.

All "mental" carbohydrate addictions can be broken in one thought. Most "physical" carbohydrate addictions are broken in a matter of four days, which is the amount of time required for insulin levels to stabilize and also for the body to eliminate most traces of the offending carbohydrate based foods. And this includes breaking most allergy addictions to heavy carbohydrates (such as sugar, corn syrup, and all sweet foods), as well as common staples (such as wheat, potatoes, oats, corn, rye, barley and other starchy grains).

Once you stop consuming high levels of carbohydrate, your body's "internal wisdom" will come to your aid and support your energy needs by developing an enzymatic network that will begin to efficiently utilize fat as fuel.[6] For most of our lives, we Americans have been burning carbohydrate and very little fat. Unless you are an endurance athlete who trains for well over one to two hours per day, "you just ain't got what it takes" to burn fat initially (and even most endurance athletes are predominantly *sugar burners* who continually *carbo load.*).

Breaking a carbohydrate addiction may require only a matter of days, but to become an efficient fat burner often requires 30-120 days, so please be patient and persevere. By following *The Fat Burning Diet* principles, your body will finally be relieved from the task of secreting high volumes of insulin each day. With the curtailment of high carbohydrate foods, your pancreas will only produce small amounts of insulin. In place of insulin, your body will secrete a powerful hormone called glucagon, which will mobilize fatty acids and begin laying the ground work for some serious fat burning activity.

The Power of Glucagon!

When blood glucose and insulin are at normal (natural) levels, glucagon pours forth from the pancreas, enters the bloodstream and signals the body to begin producing enzymes that will mobilize fat from the cells to be burned as fuel. This process is a little more complex than as described but I promised to keep this simple. Insulin is trickling into the bloodstream in minuscule amounts, while glucagon is gushing forth to conquer those fat cells and drive them out of hiding and into your metabolic furnace to be ignited as premium fuel (energy). And no hiding places can elude the "eagle eyes" of the all mighty GLUCAGON! Cellulite (rhymes with smell your feet) doesn't stand a chance against the triglycerides torching power of glucagon. Nor does a double chin, love handles, beer bellies, bubble buns, lumpy legs, or thunder thighs.

Eicosanoids, Your Fat Burning Friends

While glucagon release is the first step to the fat mobilization process, the production of another group of hormones called eicosanoids are the real secret to fat burning. By limiting the release of insulin through the control of dietary carbohydrate, the body will create a network of *friendly* eicosanoids that accelerates the use of stored bodyfat.[7] The essential fatty acids of the body are the building blocks for eicosanoid production while insulin is the controlling mechanism that determines if *friendly, fat burning* eicosanoids are to be created.

Insulin Stops Fat Burning

High levels of insulin stop the production of *friendly* eicosanoids, hence fat burning is totally dependent upon maintaining low levels of insulin in the bloodstream. How is this possible? Limit the type and amount of carbohydrate that is eaten at each meal and consume foods that are high in protein and both essential fatty acids. Eicosanoids are created within the body exclusively from the essential fatty acids, and especially from linolenic acid (flax seed oil contains approximately 57-60% linolenic acid and is one of the richest sources known. More on flax seed oil in a later chapter).

You're In Control!

Following *The Fat Burning Diet* is the ideal method for breaking even the toughest carbohydrate addiction. By eating a special balance of protein, fat and carbohydrate, your system will consistently produce the necessary hormones to keep you in the fat burning zone. And you control it all!

Chapter 5

Fat Burning Principles

The purpose of this book is to offer to the world a fat burning program that is easy to understand, simple to perform and down right fun to follow. The fat burning process can be quite boring and technical when explained in great detail. My last intent is to "turn off" my readers by dragging them through a long, detailed chapter filled with tongue twisting words, technical jargon and medical facts. To keep this book light, lively and flowing, I'll explain the fat burning process in simple, easy to understand terms.

1. To facilitate fat burning, the release of the hormone insulin must be controlled by restricting daily carbohydrate intake to a range that does not exceed 20-25% of your daily calorie needs. This range could be somewhere between 40-150 grams of carbohydrate per day, depending on total body weight and your physical activity level.

2. The type of carbohydrate must be of a nature that slowly enters the bloodstream, causing insulin to be released in very small amounts that only trickle into the bloodstream. Non-starchy vegetables are ideal carbohydrates to consume for this purpose, as well as nuts, seeds and low carbohydrate fruits.

3. An adequate amount of complete protein must accompany each meal to feed the muscles during the fat burning process, thus avoiding muscle atrophy (shrinking). If you stopped eating altogether for several days, your body would

burn fat, but it would also burn protein (which means sacrificing lean muscle) at a rate of 2/3 protein to only 1/3 fat! When we restrict carbohydrate, and maintain adequate protein intake, the body burns nearly 100% fat and almost no muscle.[8]

4. A healthy and natural source of fat must be eaten at each meal. None of that non-fat, non-sense on *The Fat Burning Diet*. Natural sources of fat are very healthy and necessary to the body. Healthy fats supply the body with essential fatty acids and help lubricate the system. Fats are also essential to buffer the release of carbohydrate into the bloodstream. When fats accompany a meal, digestion is slowed and glucose enters the blood very gradually thus requiring only a smidgen of insulin to be released that trickles into the bloodstream. Healthy fat eaten with a meal also satisfies hunger for longer periods of time, which means you will eat less *and* less often.

5. Once insulin release is curtailed by limiting the amount and type of carbohydrate consumed, the body mobilizes other insulin antagonist hormones, namely glucagon which is a fat mobilizer. Insulin is a fat maker and glucagon is a fat taker. Once the insulin tap is turned down, the body begins to create a chain of fat burning enzymes, which is a process requiring approximately 30-120 days to build this chain into an effective fat burning network.

6. Exercise speeds the fat burning process because: (a) exercise helps control carbohydrate uptake by burning any excess glucose as fuel before insulin levels rise and shut off the fat burning hormone glucagon, and (b) the more calories you burn, the more fat you burn (while following *The Fat Burning Diet* principles). It's as simple as that! Sugar burners must first burn all their presently formed glucose, then their glycogen stores and finally they get to metabolize fat. To accomplish the aforementioned process requires well over one full hour of

performing an aerobic style of exercise **before** you even get to the fat burning phase, which is an unlikely feat for the average American to adhere to on a consistent basis. On *The Fat Burning Diet* you simply burn fat. That's it!

7. Our dietary objective is to eat small amounts of carbohydrate, coupled with ample protein and wholesome fats and oils. The above combination of nutrients will keep a person on the edge of a physical state which is medically termed as ketosis/lypolisis. The body will go into a state of "ketosis" whenever carbohydrates are severely restricted, thus leaving the body no choice but to select fat as its energy source.

It is ideal to eat just enough carbohydrates to avoid being in constant ketosis, because: a) the brain requires glucose to function properly, at least until it becomes efficient at burning fat as "ketone bodies"; b) people remain of *cheery spirits* if small amounts of carbohydrates are eaten; c) no carbohydrates, or at least 0-30 grams per day, can create a gloomy outlook, especially during the transition period as a person's body is creating its fat burning network of enzymes; d) ultra low carbohydrate dieting crowds out vegetables, nuts, seeds and fruit, all of which are loaded with nutrients your body needs. e) ketosis blocks the mobilization of the fat burning hormone glucagon and initially causes some loss of muscle mass[9], until the body becomes efficient at burning "ketone bodies".

Ketosis/lypolisis is the medical name given to the fat burning process. In the diabetic, this happens unnaturally when insulin is too weak and/or not being produced. Blood sugar levels rise and, without insulin, the body is unable to utilize the excess glucose for energy, so it automatically chooses fatty acids as its energy source. If blood sugar levels are not in excess, ketosis is not harmful to the system. In fact, ketosis is actually a very energizing state of being, if a person is efficient at burning fat. Primitive Eskimos are almost always in ketosis because their diet is extremely low in carbohydrates. Ketone bodies are created within the body as it breaks down bodyfat into pairings of two carbon compounds. "Ketones" are thus a newer fatty acid, shorter in chain length by two carbon fragments which enter the metabolic pool to be used as fuel.[10]

In layman's terms, your body will select fat as energy through a seemingly complex, yet simple process. Your body merely secretes the hormone glucagon (on a low carbohydrate diet) which mobilizes fatty acids in the adipose tissue to be used as fuel, or your body creates "ketones" (on an extremely low carbohydrate diet) to burn as needed for energy and lypolisis (i.e. fat burning) takes place as a result. The consumption of excess carbohydrate, combined with a lack of physical motion, are the two main obstacles that stand in the way of these natural, metabolic processes.

8. Testing for ketosis is easy for the beginning fat burner. Simply restrict your daily carbohydrate intake to a point where the body begins to burn ketone bodies, which is usually somewhere around 25-50 grams per day (with all the carbohydrates being divided evenly between 3-4 meals). Purchase a bottle of Ketostix from your local pharmacy and begin testing your urine with the sticks. If the stick turns purple then you are in a state of ketosis, but you are not burning the ketone bodies efficiently. What has happened is your body has created ketone bodies to be used as premium fuel. Your system does not yet possess the enzymatic capacity to burn the ketones efficiently, so they spill over into your urine as waste, thus turning the Ketostix purple.

Within 30-120 days of following *The Fat Burning Diet* your body should become efficient at burning ketones, and the Ketostix will no longer turn purple no matter how low your carbohydrate intake. Your body will be adapted to readily burn ketones as fuel so virtually none remain as unburned waste. This means you are an efficient fat burner and will do well on the edge of ketosis (which is where you will be the most comfortable) or in complete ketosis (which can become very uncomfortable, especially for the first 14-21 days of consuming very low carbohydrate meals.).

9. The brain of a carbohydrate burner is dependent upon glucose as its primary source of fuel, while the brain of a fat burner is capable of utilizing ketones or glucose.[11]

10. The only physical act that blocks your body's ability to select fat as fuel is the ingestion of excess carbohydrate. You, and only you, control what foods are placed in your mouth.

Your Heart Burns Fat Exclusively!

Did you know that your heart uses FAT exclusively as its source of energy?[12] Now why would your heart only choose fat? It cannot miss a beat and needs a very reliable and optimum source of energy. Carbohydrates and glucose are too unreliable for your heart. Glucose is inferior for muscle power and only your brain is truly efficient at burning glucose as its source of fuel. Your brain is unique because it has the ability to utilize glucose without insulin being present. What this tells us is that the human body is a fat burning organism that is designed to operate on small amounts of insulin and carbohydrate.

Chapter 6

The Fat Burning Diet

*"There is absolutely no way you can **fail** on The Fat Burning Diet, because **failure** is not on the menu."*

To begin accessing fat for fuel, each individual must consume meals that are balanced with a certain amount and specific type of protein, fat and carbohydrate. Each facet in this nutrient equation is vitally important, with the amount and type of carbohydrate being the most critical aspect to control. To put it bluntly, too many "carbs" combined with limited physical activity means, "Here's the Beef!"

Do you happen to know what type of foods cattle are fed prior to their trip **to** the market? GRAINS (high carbs), which really make them fat, sassy and worth much more, because they are sold by the pound. And what do Americans eat following their trip **from** the market? GRAINS (high carbs). Now don't that just knock your hat in the crick?

The Fat Burning Diet is so simple to follow, even a small child could manage (and this diet is great for kids!) Basically there are no "nevers" in the diet plan (I like that idea!). This diet offers flexibility to suit your individual needs and desires. Also, once per week you may go out or stay home and eat anything you desire. What this actually means is that during one meal per week, you may unhinge your belt, slide back your sleeves, strap on the feed bag and boogie! This is a no-holds-barred, all you can hold down, see-food disappearing act! And the time limit for this dining match is one 60 minute round per week, period! At the end of 60 minutes I want a clean break! That means drop the shovel, push back that cherry cheese cake topped with deep fried cheese balls and come up for air! Besides, there is always next week.

I'll bet you love my diet already, don't you? In fact, I'm such a great guy I'll even let you begin *The Fat Burning Diet* with your once a week all you can eat "wang dang doodle" meal (remember Savoy Brown?). You don't have to start it that way, but you can if you wish. But after your 60 minute "free-for-all" you will begin your next meal by utilizing *The Fat Burning Diet* principles (and I don't want any ifs, ands or bubble butts!).

With the flexibility aspect behind us now (don't look back), let's dive in and start torching those triglycerides! *The Fat Burning Diet* is going to help you "melt away" fat fast. Actually fat burns and doesn't really "melt" *away*, so don't worry. You won't be at a party with a big puddle forming at your feet, or anything like that.

The Fat Burning Diet is offered in three unique levels of Melting Power: *Mini-Burn*, *Mega-Burn* and *Maxi-Burn*, each designed to suite your own individual tastes and desired outcome. The *Mini-Burn* plan may be used as a stepping stone or you may simply dive in wherever you wish and start "burning!" Some days you may desire to mix and match by eating a *Mini-Burn* breakfast, *Mega-Burn* lunch and a *Maxi-Burn* dinner.

The Mini-Burn Plan

This is a great way to begin *The Fat Burning Diet*. Being higher in healthy fats, the diet and menu suggestions are deeply satisfying and especially effective when employed to break away from carbohydrate dependency. This diet plan is also very effective for bodybuilders, powerlifters and strength athletes who are training hard and desire to gain lean mass.

The Mega-Burn Plan

Being moderate in fat and balanced in protein and carbohydrate, the *Mega-Burn Plan* is easy to follow and produces a slow steady burn. Utilizing naturally occurring amounts of healthy fats, this diet plan is fit for a king and performs well in the *long haul.* Once you become an efficient fat burner, many of your meals will probably be selected from this menu category.

The Maxi-Burn Plan

If it's ultra low bodyfat you desire, or you are a competitive athlete or just someone who loves to "burn it to the max", then The *Maxi-Burn Plan* is for you. Competitive bodybuilders thrive on this diet plan! Centered around lowfat protein sources, coupled with small amounts of healthy fats, and precisely the right amount of carbohydrate to make you "sizzle", this unique plan will bring out those elusive abdominals in men and keep the ladies trim, tight and out of sight!

Special Note: Before beginning *The Fat Burning Diet,* it is advisable that you:
1. Discuss the program with your doctor of choice and receive a medical check-up, especially if you have any health problems.
2. Have a blood test performed to determine your present lipid ratios (cholesterol, HDL, LDL, VLDL and triglycerides). Follow-up blood tests should be performed every 2-3 months after beginning the program to note any changes in your fat profile.
3. Weigh yourself and measure your bodyfat levels, then record and date these figures in a special notebook.
4. Select a bodyfat percentage goal for yourself that you are positive you can achieve. If, for example, your initial

bodyfat measurement is 23%, then try to reach 21% in 30 days and 19% in 60 days, etc. DO NOT RELY ON THE SCALE ALONE FOR FEED-BACK! Scales only tell if you have lost or gained weight, not fat. Sometimes you gain muscle as you lose fat, so the scale might not show any change at all, which can be very deceiving unless you are tracking your bodyfat percentages.

5. Post the following affirmation on your bedroom or bathroom mirror, or somewhere that you will see it and then read it every day: *"Fat is my friend and is here to serve me with endless energy to reach my goals and beyond. Life has all its doors open to me and I am committed to succeed in all my endeavors. I am willing to do what ever it takes to make my dreams become reality."*

"There is no such thing as one set diet plan. Eating is an ever changing process that fluctuates daily to meet one's needs, tastes, desires and availability of food."

The Fat Burning Diet's Four Food Groups

Food Group I
Proteins: Chicken, fish, turkey, beef, meats, eggs, cottage cheese, cheese, plain yogurt, desiccated liver tablets, egg white protein powders (no carbohydrates added), milk and egg white protein powders (no carbohydrates added), Amino acids capsules (complete amino acid formulas, not isolated aminos).

Food Group II
Non-Starchy Vegetables: Artichokes, asparagus, beets, beans (yellow wax or green), bean sprouts, cabbage (all varieties) carrots, cauliflower, celery, chives, corn, cucumbers, dandelion greens, eggplant, endive. escarole, garlic, green peas, kale, kohl rabi, leeks,

lettuce (all varieties), mustard greens, okra, onions, parsnips, peppers (green, red, jalapeno, Anaheim, etc.), radishes, shallots, spinach, string beans, squash (summer varieties only), Swiss chard, tomatoes, turnips, turnip greens, watercress.

Food Group III
Fresh Fruits: Apples, apricots, avocados, ripe bananas, blueberries, cantaloupe, cherries, cranberries, figs, grapefruit, grapes, kumquats, lemons, limes, mangoes, melons (all varieties), nectarines, oranges, papaya, peaches, pears, pineapple, persimmons, plums, raspberries, strawberries, watermelon.

Food Group IV
*"Friendly" Fats and Oils: Flax seed oil, olive oil, almonds, brazil nuts, filberts, pecans, pine nuts, walnuts, raw cream, raw butter, lecithin granules and the naturally occurring fats found in meat, eggs and dairy products.

* "Friendly" fats and oils are healthy fatty acids present in olives, nuts, seeds, wholesome meats (chicken, fish, turkey, etc.). "Unhealthy" fats and oils are heat processed, deep fried, hydrogenated (margarine and vegetable shortening are both hydrogenated oils, meaning they have been pressed with hydrogen to make them solid at room temperature), and rancid, refined oils, as are found on most supermarket shelves. "Healthy" oils must usually be purchased at a natural food grocery store. The one healthy oil that can be found in any supermarket is pure, virgin olive oil, thanks to the Italian Americans!

The Fat Burning Diet "No-Nos"

1. No sugar, candy, sugary sodas, juice, sugary or sweet desserts, jelly, cookies or other sweet foods. And this includes hidden sugars found in ketchup, salad dressings and all packaged and canned foods. READ ALL LABELS VERY CARE-

FULLY!

2. No milk of any type including skim, 2%, whole, raw, etc. (milk is high in a sugar known as lactose).

3. No wheat. This includes bread, pasta, gravies, buns, breading, stuffing, etc.

4. No barley malt, brown sugar, honey, glucose, lactose, glucose polymers, concentrated grape juice, fructose, energy drinks, energy type candy bars, or endurance drinks.

5. No hydrogenated oils, processed oils, fried foods or margarine.

6. No beans (dried varieties) including: Pinto, black, navy, great northern, adzuki, etc. (green or waxed beans are OK).

7. No salt and salted foods including: Potato chips, crackers, pretzels, canned goods or any other food that is laced with sodium. Read all labels. (salt can cause bloating, water retention and is a contributing factor to over eating).

8. No processed meats including: bacon; bologna; hot dogs; sausage; lunch meat and all smoked meats (unless naturally processed and chemical free).

9. No starchy foods including: potatoes; yams; sweet potatoes; winter squash; barley; brown rice; buckwheat; corn tortillas; millet; rye; and corn bread. (note: While not optimum for burning fat, starches may be used occasionally if they are limited to 10-25 grams of total carbohydrate per meal. Whole food starches, except wheat, are allowed just for menu variety, especially during transition from a carbohydrate burner to a fat burner).

10. No fructose or anything it is added to including protein powders, soft drinks, sports drinks, fluid replacers, etc. Fructose is low on the glycemic chart, meaning that it enters the bloodstream very slowly which helps to limit the insulin response. Sounds like a fat burner's dream come true? Wrong! There is still a substantial insulin response with fructose as an isolated sweetener, plus fructose has been found to significantly elevate triglycerides and LDL (low density "transporter" lipoproteins) levels, while lowering HDL (high density "retriever" lipoproteins) levels.[13]

11. No snacks between meals. If you desire to eat a small meal instead of a large one, then make it a balanced, fat burning meal and not an unbalanced between-meal snack.

12. No alcoholic beverages should be consumed, except for an occasional 2-3 ounce glass of dry wine with a meal. Alcohol is a unique carbohydrate that requires virtually no digestion and can pass directly through the stomach wall to enter the bloodstream. Part of the "high", from drinking alcoholic beverages, is the "blood sugar rush" that one experiences when glucose levels in the bloodstream rise very rapidly. But what goes up, must come down. High blood sugar levels are simply the prerequisite for bodyfat formation. Do yourself a big fat burning favor and severely limit all alcohol consumption.

Enough of the" No-Nos. "
Here are The Fat Burning Diet "Yes-Yesses"

1. Yes, eat ample amounts of complete proteins from Food Group I.

2. Yes, eat a wide variety of fresh vegetables, from Food Group II, preferably raw in the form of salads.

3. Yes, use 1-3 tbs. of fresh flax seed oil daily. Flax oil is wonderful in protein drinks and as a salad dressing (see the recipe section in Chapter 17).

4. Yes, eat raw nuts and seeds occasionally to receive their special blend of essential fatty acids, vitamins and minerals. Soak them for 24 hours in water to improve their digestibility.

5. Yes, drink plenty of pure water. Fat burning is a dehydrating process that requires ample quantities of water. Your daily water needs could be anywhere from 1 quart to 1 gallon, depending on climate and your body weight. How to know you are getting enough? Drink water when you are thirsty, and drink enough to keep your urine light in color.

6. Yes, eat 3-5 small to medium size meals daily. At each meal consume a balance of protein, fat and carbohydrate, approximately as follows: 30-55% protein, 15-20% carbohydrate, 25-55% fat (healthy fats only). These meal percentages (depending on the size of the individual and their activity or fitness level) equate to approximately 25-80 grams of protein, 10-40 grams of carbohydrate, 10-50 grams of healthy fats and oils.

7. Yes, eat your 3-5 meals in a 12 hour period, followed by a period of no food for the next 12 hour period. This will greatly improve your digestion and elimination. What this means is that you can "chow down" as late as 6:00-7:00 PM. and then nothing more until 6:00-7:00 am. If you ate at midnight, then nothing the next day until the "crack of noon."

8. Yes, use a protein supplement if necessary to be consistent with your meal times and balance. Do not buy any of the typical protein powders on the market. Read all labels carefully, and I mean the fine print! Most protein powders are laced with cheap carbohydrate fillers that immediately move you from the fat burning mode into the fat storing mode. Select a pure egg white, or milk and egg white formula that contains only protein, with no fat and no more than one gram of carbohydrate per twenty four grams of protein per one ounce serving.

Athletes Need More Protein!

The protein controversy has gone on for years, but recent research has indicated an increased need for protein by athletes, especially strength athletes, bodybuilders, power lifters and football players.[14] In general, anyone lifting weights that wishes to grow more muscle should be eating, on a daily basis, approximately one gram to one and a half grams of complete protein per pound of *lean* body weight. For all endurance athletes, 2/3 to 3/4 gram of protein per pound of lean body weight is usually plenty. These are not exact figures, but very good estimations.

If you are sedentary, your protein (and calorie) needs are usually much less than someone who is lifting weights, running, biking or active in sports. A sedentary individual may do just fine on 1/2 gram of complete protein per pound of lean body weight. *The Fat Burning Diet* encourages ACTIVITY, so if you are "a sedentary kind of person", then be prepared to increase your protein intake as you increase your motion.

The Vital Importance of Raw Foods

Enzymes (not bread) are the "staff" of life, controlling literally thousands of known and unknown functions in the human body. Enzymes are protein molecules that carry the *forces of life* within them.[15] Without enzymes we could not exist. Fat burning is controlled by enzymes, as is digestion, elimination, and countless other internal functions. Enzymes are very fragile and are destroyed by heat.

All *raw* foods (foods that are uncooked or unheated beyond a temperature of 125-130 degrees Fahrenheit) contain enzymes. All *cooked* foods (foods that have been heated for a certain period of time above the temperature of 130 degrees Fahrenheit) have all of their enzymatic activity destroyed by the intense heat.

It is interesting to note that the human being is the only creature on earth that cooks their food. All other life forms simply eat their food raw and unheated (unless humans have intervened with their eating habits as in the case of domestic animals or animals held captive in parks and zoos). I've never seen a raccoon broiling its dinner or a lion at a barbecue or a rabbit steaming its garden veggies. All animals find their daily food and eat it as is.

Because *The Fat Burning Diet* eliminates or severely restricts cooked starchy foods, the door is opened for plenty of raw foods including: vegetables; fruits; flax seed oil; nuts and seeds. And these raw foods are vitally important to our health and well being.

The typical American diet is often deficient in raw food enzymes. In fact, with the exception of a few vegetable salads and an occasional piece of fruit, many Americans rarely ever eat raw foods. Cooked foods that are common to the diet of most humans are: all breads; pasta; potatoes; yams; squash; roasted nuts including peanuts; peanut butter; jelly; crackers; cookies; candy bars; all meats; eggs; tofu; steamed vegetables; gravy; canned goods; frozen foods; packaged foods; ice cream; pies; cakes; candy; chips; and all dairy products including cheese; milk; yogurt; cottage cheese; cream; half and half (unless they are unpasteurized, which we have the option of buying in California).

Are you beginning to get the idea of just how many of our foods are cooked, dead and lifeless? On *The Fat Burning Diet* you will be eating a high percentage of your foods raw.

NOTE: Eating raw meat, fish, poultry, eggs and dairy products would truly be the ultimate on *The Fat Burning Diet*, but is not advisable due to parasites in many protein foods, the general poor health of the animals and the difficulty in obtaining truly fresh foods that are not spoiled or contaminated. Because of the above reasons, it is best to **only consume raw foods that are not of animal origin,** with the exception of *raw* dairy products in states where they are available and carefully monitored.

Chapter 7

Fat Burning Menu Ideas

Weekly Fat Burning Diet Menus.

For fat burning to be a part of your life, consistency must become a main constituent of your daily meals. You can not burn fat by eating haphazardly, nor can you *sizzle* that adipose tissue by missing a meal and "loading-up" on the next one.

Listed below are the three weekly menu plans for burning fat: *The Mini-Burn Plan*, *The Mega-Burn Plan* and *The Maxi-Burn Plan*.

Making Menu Adjustments To Meet Your Specific Needs

Approximate amounts listed are for an active, 160 lb. (lean weight) athletic male that lifts weights. Make menu adjustments according to your weight and activity level. A 235 lb. construction worker will obviously need many more calories than a 100 lb. secretary. Merely increase or decrease total calories of the menus to suite your needs, keeping the proper ratio of Protein to Carbohydrate to Fat (P-C-F ratio) balance of 30-55% protein, 15-20% carbohydrate and 25-55% fats and oils.

Accurate menu adjustments may be accomplished by multiplying or dividing the portions of each menu suggestion to achieve the increase or decrease of calories you desire.

Example: A very active woman that weighs 150 lb. with 20% bodyfat, actually possesses 120 lb. of lean tissue and 30 lb. of fat. (total weight minus bodyfat). To adjust the menu suggestions to meet her general needs, all portions of the meals would merely need to be multiplied by approximately 75% (160 times 75% equals

120). Six ounces of tuna would become four ounces and one apple would become 3/4 of an apple, etc.

If you weigh 200 lb. lean, then simply multiply by 125% for each portion. (160 times 125% equals 200). If you are an extremely active person, then increase all portions an extra 5-10%. If you are sedentary, then decrease total calories by 5-10% to meet your needs. With a little trial and error, you will discover your perfect balance.

The key to the success of this diet program is to control the amount and type of carbohydrate you are consuming, thus keeping insulin's release to a trickle, which automatically stimulates the body to naturally burn fat, all day and all night long. You will be burning both dietary fat and bodyfat as fuel, so ample quantities of *natural* dietary fat will be important as a valuable source of premium fuel.

Mini-Burn 7 Day Menu Ideas (little sizzle)
P-C-F ratio target zone: 30% protein; 20% carbohydrate; 50% healthy fat and oils.

Day 1:

Meal 1
4 egg omelet, 2 ounces of cheese, 1 med. apple, 3 ounces water packed tuna.
Calories: 746   Protein: 61 grams   Carbohydrate: 35 grams
Fat: 40 grams
Protein to Carbohyrate to Fat calorie percentage ratio: 33-19-49

Meal 2
Large salad, 1 tablespoon. olive oil, squeeze of lemon, 4 ounces water packed tuna, 2 ounces cheese, 20 grapes.
Calories: 602   Protein: 46 grams   Carbohydrate: 30 grams
Fat: 35 grams
P-C-F ratio: 30-19-50

Meal 3
Mini-Burn Protein Drink(see Recipes, Chapter 17).

Meal 4
Small salad, 2 tablespoons dressing of choice (see recipes), 6 ounce beef patty, 4 ounces green beans, 1 medium apple.
Calories: 711   Protein: 52 grams   Carbohydrates: 34 grams
Fat: 41 grams
P-C-F ratio: 29-19-52

Day 2:

Meal 1
6 ounces lo-fat cottage cheese, 1 tablespoon flax seed oil, 5 straw-berries, 2 scrambled eggs.
Calories: 516   Protein: 38 grams   Carbohydrate: 30 grams
Fat: 28 grams
P-C-F ratio: 29-23-48

Meal 2
Small salad, 1 tablespoon olive oil, 4 ounces baked, skinless chicken breast, 6 ounces steamed zucchini topped with 1 tablespoon sour cream, 1 medium peach.
Calories: 484   Protein 39 grams   Carbohydrate: 25 grams
Fat: 26 grams
P-C-F ratio: 32-20-48

Meal 3
Two slices of "Banana Dream Pie" (see Recipes, Chapter 17).
Calories: 442   Protein: 34 grams   Carbohydrate: 9 grams
Fat: 27 grams
P-C-F ratio: 30-17-54

Meal 4
Small salad, 1 tablespoon dressing, 6 ounces broiled fish, 1 small
yam, 2 ounces cheese.
Calories: 781   Protein: 60 grams   Carbohydrate: 40 grams
Fat: 42 grams
P-C-F ratio: 31-21-48

Day 3:

Meal 1
Cheese and Spinach Omelet (4 eggs, 1 ounce cheese, 1 ounce
chopped spinach), 1 orange, 4 ounces lo-fat yogurt.
Calories: 548   Protein: 40 grams   Carbohydrate: 26 grams
Fat: 32 grams
P-C-F ratio: 29-19-52

Meal 2
Mini-Burn Protein Drink (see Recipes, Chapter 17)

Meal 3
Small salad, 1/4 cup almonds, 3 hard boiled eggs, 1/2 cup cooked
brown rice, 3 ounces water packed tuna.
Calories: 664   Protein: 51 grams   Carbohydrate: 36 grams
Fat: 35 grams
P-C-F ratio: 31-21-48

Meal 4
1/2 cup steamed cauliflower, 2 ounces grated cheese, 4 ounces
extra lean beef patty, 1 small papaya.
Calories: 661   Protein: 50 grams   Carbohydrate: 34 grams
Fat: 37 grams
P-C-F ratio: 30-20-50

Day 4

Meal 1
Protein Drink (see Recipes, Chapter 17).

Meal 2
6 ounces cottage cheese topped with: 1 small diced apple, 2 ounces of shelled walnuts, 1 tablespoon "natural" whipped cream (see recipes) and sprinkled with cinnamon; 3 ounces turkey breast.
Calories: 835   Protein: 64 grams   Carbohydrates: 40 grams
Fat: 50 grams
P-C-F ratio: 30-19-51

Meal 3
Large salad, 2 tablespoons dressing, 2 ounces cheese, 6 ounces broiled fish, 1 peach.
Calories: 697   Protein: 60 grams   Carbohydrate: 20 grams
Fat: 42 grams
P-C-F ratio: 35-12-54

Meal 4
Large chef salad containing: a variety of fresh vegetables, 6 ounces of chopped chicken, 1/4 avocado (diced), 1 ounce chopped walnuts, 2 tablespoons dressing, 20 grapes.
Calories: 821   Protein: 57 grams   Carbohydrate: 36 grams
Fat: 52 grams
P-C-F ratio: 27-17-56

Day 5

Meal 1
2 ounces raw almonds, 6 ounces lo-fat plain yogurt, 2 scrambled eggs, 3 ounces chicken breast, 8 strawberries.
Calories: 806   Protein: 61 grams   Carbohydrate: 43 grams

Fat: 46 grams
P-C-F ratio: 29-21-50

Meal 2
Protein drink of choice (see Recipes, Chapter17).

Meal 3
6 ounces extra lean hamburger patty topped with onion slices and 2 ounces cheese, 1 orange, 4 ounces steamed green beans topped with 1 ounce chopped almonds.
Calories: 950   Protein: 72 grams   Carbohydrate: 33 grams
Fat: 61 grams ,
P-C-F ratio: 30-14-56

Meal 4
4 ounces chicken, 2 ounces steamed broccoli, small salad with 2 ounces dressing, 2 ounces grated cheese, 1 medium apple.
Calories: 684   Protein: 50 grams   Carbohydrate:30 grams
Fat: 42 grams
P-C-F ratio: 29-17-54

Day 6

Meal 1
4 egg omelet with 2 ounces cheese (topped with 2 tablespoons salsa and green pepper slices), 1 ounce raw almonds, 1 medium apple.
Calories: 779   Protein: 45 grams   Carbohydrate: 31 grams
Fat: 54 grams
P-C-F ratio: 23-16-61

Meal 2
4 egg spinach omelet with 2 ounces cheese, 6 ounces plain yogurt, 10 strawberries.
Calories: 728   Protein: 47 grams   Carbohydrate: 34 grams

Fat: 45 grams
P-C-F ratio: 26-19-56

Meal 3
6 ounces lean beef patty, 2 cups mixed salad, 4 cucumber slices, 1 tablespoon flax seed oil, 1 nectarine.
Calories: 722   Protein: 54 grams   Carbohydrate: 32 grams
Fat: 43 grams
P-C-F ratio: 30-17-53

Meal 4
6 ounces water packed tuna, 1/2 ripe avocado (diced) over a small vegetable salad, 1 cup cantaloupe cubes.
Calories: 602   Protein: 50 grams   Carbohydrate: 33 grams
Fat: 33 grams
P-C-F ratio: 32-21-47

Day 7

Meal 1
6 ounces whole milk plain yogurt topped with 1/2 cup blueberries, 1 tablespoon Natural Whipped Cream (see Recipes, Chapter 17), 2 poached eggs, 2 ounces turkey breast.
Calories: 459   Protein: 38 grams   Carbohydrate: 22 grams
Fat: 24 grams
P-C-F ratio: 33-20-47

Meal 2
Protein drink of choice (see Recipes, Chapter 17).

Meal 3
Taco salad containing: 6 ounces extra lean beef over 1 cup of

mixed salad, topped with sour cream, 2 tablespoons salsa, 1 chopped tomato and 2 ounces grated cheese.
Calories: 809   Protein: 68 grams   Carbohydrate: 23 grams
Fat: 50 grams
P-C-F ratio: 33-11-55

Meal 4
Large chef salad topped with 4 ounces water packed tuna, 2 ounces cheese, 1 tablespoon flax seed oil, 2 kiwi fruit for dessert.
Calories: 654   Protein: 48 grams   Carbohydrate: 36 grams
Fat: 36 grams
P-C-F ratio: 29-23-48

Each of the above menu ideas contain ample amounts of "friendly" (healthy) fats and oils, which are very satisfying to the appetite, making them ideal for transitioning from a high carbohydrate diet to *The Fat Burning Diet*. Once a carbohydrate addiction is broken and fat burning is underway, you may desire to choose your meals from the lower fat, lower calorie *Mega-Burn* or *Maxi-Burn* menu suggestions. Transition periods may range from 30 days to six months depending upon the person and their present state of health and level of fitness. Feeling a steady flow of energy all day long, combined with the absence of any carbohydrate cravings is a good sign that it's time to move on to the *Mega-Burn* or *Maxi-Burn* menu ideas.

Bodybuilders, powerlifters and strength athletes may utilize the *Mini-Burn Plan* to gain lean mass. One or two extra protein drinks per day may also be added to increase calorie and protein requirements. Following one to two years on the *Mini-Burn Plan*, the strength athlete may then desire to shift over to the *Mega-Burn Plan* to get even leaner while maintaining the muscle mass he or she developed from lifting heavy weights and following the *Mini-Burn Plan*.

Mega-Burn 7 Day Menu Ideas (super sizzle)
P-F-C ratio target zone: 40% protein; 20% carbohydrate; 40% fat.

Day 1

Meal 1
4 egg whites - 3 yolks, 3 ounces chicken breast, 1 small peach.
Calories: 421   Protein: 49 grams   Carbohydrate: 12 grams
Fat: 18 grams
P-C-F ratio: 48-12-40

Meal 2
2 cups salad, 1 tablespoons flax seed oil, squeeze of lemon, 6 ounces turkey breast, 20 grapes.
Calories: 607   Protein: 53 grams   Carbohydrate: 34 grams
Fat: 29 grams
P-C-F ratio: 35-22-43

Meal 3
Mega-Burn protein drink (see Recipes, Chapter 17).

Meal 4
2 cups salad, 1 tablespoon flax seed oil, 6 ounces chicken, 4 ounces blueberries, 1 hard boiled egg.
Calories: 667   Protein: 60 grams   Carbohyrate: 32 grams
Fat: 34 grams
P-C-F ratio: 36-19-45

Day 2

Meal 1
8 ounces low-fat cottage cheese, 1 tablespoon flax seed oil, 6 strawberries, 3 egg whites-1 yolk.
Calories: 498   Protein: 46 grams   Carbohydrate: 23 grams

Fat: 24 grams
P-C-F ratio: 37-19-44

Meal 2
Small salad, 1 tablespoon dressing, 6 ounces tuna (water packed),
1 ounce cheese, 4 ounce banana.
Calorie: 532   Protein: 53 grams   Carbohydrate: 25 grams
Fat: 25 grams
P-C-F ratio: 39-19-42

Meal 3
Mega-Burn protein drink (see Recipes. Chapter 17)

Meal 4
1/2 cup cantaloupe (eaten first), 2 cups salad, 1 tablespoon flax
oil, 6 ounces fresh fish (broiled).
Calories: 466   Protein: 46 grams   Carbohydrate: 17 grams
Fat: 24 grams
P-C-F ratio: 40-14-46

Day 3

Meal 1
Protein drink of choice (see Recipes, Chapter 17).

Meal 2
6 egg whites, 3 yolks, 1 small apple, 3 ounces turkey breast.
Calories: 524   Protein: 54 grams   Carbohydrate: 24 grams
Fat: 22 grams
P-C-F ratio: 42-19-39

Meal 3
1 cup salad, 6 ounces extra lean beef patty, 1 and 1/2 cups cubed

honeydew.
Calories: 564   Protein: 51 grams   Carbohydrate: 28 grams
Fat: 28 grams
P-C-F ratio: 36-20-44

Meal 4

1 cup small salad, 1 tablespoon olive oil, 4 ounces steamed green beans, 4 egg white omelet with 2 yolks, 3 ounces chicken breast, 1/2 mango.
Calories: 571   Protein: 50 grams   Carbohydrate: 33 grams
Fat: 27 grams
P-C-F ratio: 35-23-43

Day 4

Meal 1

2 ounces cheese, 6 ounces turkey breast, 1 and 1/2 cups of fresh pineapple cubes.
Calories: 671   Protein: 64 grams   Carbohydrate: 30 grams
Fat: 33 grams
P-F-C ratio: 38-18-44

Meal 2

Large chef salad containing: raw vegetables of choice, 1/4 ripe avocado (diced), 6 ounces chopped chicken, 2 tablepsoons dressing, 1 medium apple.
Calories: 683   Protein: 54 grams   Carbohydrate: 39 grams
Fat: 36 grams
P-C-F ratio: 31-22-46

Meal 3

1 cup salad (no dressing), 6 ounces lean beef patty, 1 medium bartlett pear.
Calories: 573   Protein: 51 grams   Carbohydrate: 30 grams

Fat: 28 grams
P-C-F ratio: 35-21-44

Meal 4
6 ounces plain lo-fat yogurt, 1 ounce chopped walnuts, 3 strawberries, 1 ounce milk and egg protein powder sprinkled over the
top and then stirred together.
Calories: 418   Protein: 38 grams   Carbohydrate: 24 grams
Fat: 21 grams
P-C-F ratio: 35-22-43

Day 5

Meal 1
4 egg whites - 2 yolks, 3 ounce turkey breast, 6 ounce plain lo-fat
yogurt topped with 12 chopped almonds, 1/2 apple (diced).
Calories: 581   Protein: 56 grams   Carbohydrate: 27 grams
Fat: 27 grams
P-C-F ratio: 39-19-42

Meal 2
Mega-Burn protein drink (see Recipes, Chapter 17)

Meal 3
12 ounces lowfat cottage cheese topped with: 1 tablespoon flax
seed oil, 1/2 cup fresh blueberries.
Calories: 581   Protein: 56 grams   Carbohydrate: 23 grams
Fat: 21 grams
P-C-F ratio: 40-19-40

Meal 4
2 cups large salad containing: fresh vegetables topped with, 6
ounces tuna (water packed), 1 hard boiled egg (sliced), 1 medium
apple (diced), 1 ounces walnut halves.

Calories: 726   Protein: 65 grams   Carbohydrate: 42 grams
Fat: 35 grams
P-C-F ratio: 35-23-42

Day 6

Meal 1
3 eggs, 1/2 cup of blueberries, 4 ounces ground turkey (broiled),
1 medium peach.
Calories: 526   Protein: 53 grams   Carbohydrate: 22 grams
Fat: 25 grams
P-C-F ratio: 41-17-42

Meal 2
Taco salad containing: 2 cups salad vegetables of choice, 5 ounces
extra lean ground beef (cooked), 1 green onion (chopped), 3 table-
spoons fresh salsa, 1 tomato (chopped), 1 ounce grated cheese,
chopped fresh cilantro to taste, 5 strawberries for dessert.
Calories: 624   Protein: 53 grams   Carbohydrate: 30 grams
Fat: 34 grams
P-C-F ratio: 33-19-48

Meal 3
Mega-Burn protein drink of choice (see Recipes, Chapter 17).

Meal 4
1 cup salad, 1 tablespoon dressing, 6 ounces turkey, 10 strawber-
ries in a bowl and covered with 2 ounces of half and half.
Calories: 576   Protein: 54 grams   Carbohydrate: 30 grams
Fat: 27 grams
P-C-F ratio: 37-21-42

Day 7

Meal 1
2 ounces lean beef patty, 1 small orange, 3 eggs.
Calories: 415   Protein: 35 grams   Carbohydrate: 23 grams
Fat: 20 grams
P-C-F ratio: 34-22-44

Meal 2
Mega-Burn protein drink of choice (see Recipes, Capter 17).

Meal 3
1 cup salad, 2 tablespoons dressing, 10 raw almonds, 5 ounces
skinless turkey breast, 1 medium apple.
Calories: 527   Protein: 48 grams   Carbohydrate: 28 grams
Fat: 26 grams
P-C-F ratio: 36-21-43

Meal 4
1 cup salad, 2 tablespoons dressing, 5 ounces tuna (water packed),
1 cup steamed zucchini, 1/2 cup Bing cherries.
Calories: 394   Protein: 40 grams   Carbohydrate: 22 grams
Fat: 17 grams
P-C-F ratio: 40-22-37

The above menu outlines provide ample proteins and a wide
variety of "friendly" (healthy) fats and naturally derived carbohydrates. You may always utilize the menu ideas in the *Mega-Burn*
category because these meals will provide you with optimum nutrition and superb fat burning activity.

Maxi-Burn 7 Day Menu Ideas (Ultra-sizzle!)
P-C-F ratio target zone: 50% protein; 20% carbohydrate; 30% fat.

Day 1

Meal 1
5 egg whites-2 yolks, *Maxi-Burn* protein drink containing 2 ounces egg white protein, 1/2 tablespoon flax seed oil, 4 ounces banana.
Calories: 569   Protein: 72 grams   Carbohydrate: 29 grams
Fat: 18 grams
P-C-F ratio: 51-20-28

Meal 2
Small salad, 1 tablespoon flax seed oil, 1 tablespoon fresh lemon juice, 8 ounces tuna (water packed).
Calories: 501   Protein: 60 grams   Carbohydrate: 27 grams
Fat: 17 grams
P-C-F ratio: 48-22-31

Meal 3
Small salad, 1 tablespoon olive oil, 1 squeeze lime, 8 ounces skinless turkey breast, 1.5 cups fresh pineapple chunks.
Calories: 642   Protein: 72 grams   Carbohydrate: 35 grams
Fat: 24 grams
P-C-F ratio: 45-22-33

Meal 4
10 raw almonds, 1 cup salad, 6 ounces swordfish (broiled), 6 ounces lo-fat cottage cheese.
Calories: 561   Protein: 71 grams   Carbohydrate: 25 grams
Fat: 19 grams
P-C-F ratio: 51-18-31

Day 2

Meal 1
8 ounces lo-fat cottage cheese, 1/2 tablespoon flax seed oil, 15 grapes, 3 ounces water packed tuna.
Calories: 418   Protein: 54 grams   Carbohydrate: 22 grams
Fat: 13 grams
P-C-F ratio: 52-21-27

Meal 2
Maxi-Burn Protein drink (see Recipes, Chapter 17).

Meal 3
1 cup salad (no dressing), 2 cups steamed green beans, 8 ounces turkey breast, and 2 cups sliced and steamed zucchini.
Calories: 583   Protein: 75 grams   Carbohydrate: 31 grams
Fat: 19 grams
P-C-F ratio: 50-21-29

Meal 4
2 cups cantaloupe cubes (eaten first), 1 cup salad, 5 egg white-2 yolk omelet with 4 ounces chopped turkey breast.
Calories: 559   Protein: 60 grams   Carbohydrate: 34 grams
Fat: 20 grams
P-C-F ratio: 43-24-33

Day 3

Meal 1
Maxi-Burn Protein drink (see Recipes, Chapter 17).

Meal 2
Salad containing: a bed of fresh vegetables, 6 ounces tuna (water packed), 1 hard boiled egg, 1 medium apple (diced), 1 tablespoon

olive oil (or 2 tablespoons dressing from Recipes, Chapter 17).
Calories: 525   Protein: 60 grams   Carbohydrate: 32 grams
Fat: 21 grams
P-C-F ratio: 40-24-36

Meal 3

1 cup mixed steamed vegetables, 1 cup lo-fat cottage cheese, 4 ounces extra lean beef patty topped with 1 tablespoon barbecue sauce.
Calories: 621   Protein: 69 grams   Carbohydrate: 34 grams
Fat: 23 grams
P-C-F ratio: 45-22-33

Meal 4

Maxi-Burn Protein drink (see Recipes, Chapter 17).

Day 4

Meal 1

6 ounces nonfat yogurt mixed with: 1/2 tablespoon flax seed oil, 1 ounce egg white protein powder, and then topped with 6 walnuts halves and one tangerine (sectioned, and sliced).
Calories: 559   Protein: 71 grams   Carbohydrate; 25 grams
Fat: 19 grams
P-C-F ratio: 51-18-31

Meal 2

2 cups salad, 1/2 tablespoon olive oil dressing, 8 ounces turkey breast, 2 kiwi fruit.
Calories: 642   Protein: 69 grams   Carbohydrate: 33 grams
Fat: 26 grams
P-C-F ratio: 43-20-36

Meal 3

1.5 cups steamed green beans, 8 ounces fresh fish, 1 carrot.

Calories: 472   Protein: 59 grams   Carbohydrate: 19 grams
Fat: 17 grams
P-C-F ratio: 50-16-33

Meal 4
6 ounces chicken breast, 1/4 avocado mashed as a dip, 6 long celery sticks (for dipping).
Calories: 385   Protein: 55 grams   Carbohydrate: 10 grams
Fat: 14 grams
P-C-F ratio: 61-8-30

Day 5

Meal 1
Maxi-Burn Protein Drink (see Recipes, Chapter 17).

Meal 2
6 ounces water packed tuna topped with 1/4 avocado, 1 cup of salad, fresh cilantro and 2 tablespoons salsa, 1/2 sweet potato.
Calories: 448   Protein: 48 grams   Carbohydrate: 27 grams
Fat: 17 grams
P-C-F ratio: 42-24-34

Meal 3
Small salad, 1/2 tablespoon flax seed oil, 6 ounces lobster tail, 1 cup steamed broccoli.
Calories: 330   Protein: 40 grams   Carbohydrate: 15 grams
Fat: 13 grams
P-C-F ratio: 47-18-35

Meal 4
1 cup salad, 1 tablespoon dressing of choice (no dressing), 3 ounces grilled beef liver, 3 ounce chicken breast, 2 cups steamed cauli-

flower.
Calories: 398   Protein: 54 grams   Carbohydrate: 22 grams
Fat: 11 grams
P-C-F ratio: 54-22-24

Day 6

Meal 1
6 egg whites-1 yolk, 3 ounces turkey breast, 6 ounces nonfat yogurt topped with 1/2 tbs. flax seed oil and 5 strawberries.
Calories: 484   Protein: 60 grams   Carbohydrate: 27 grams
Fat: 14 grams
P-C-F ratio: 50-23-27

Meal 2
1 cup small salad, 8 ounces swordfish, 2 cups steamed broccoli.
Calories: 465   Protein: 57 grams   Carbohydrate: 23 grams
Fat: 18 grams
P-C-F ratio: 47-19-33

Meal 3
2 cups cottage cheese, 3 ounces chicken breast, 1 Valencia orange.
Calories: 631   Protein: 80 grams   Carbohydrate: 26 grams
Fat: 22 grams
P-C-F ratio: 51-16-32

Meal 4
6 ounces water packed tuna, 4 stalks celery, 1 carrot, 1/2 avocado.
Calories: 416   Protein: 47 grams   Carbohydrate: 21 grams
Fat: 17 grams
P-C-F ratio: 44-20-36

Day 7

Meal 1
6 egg whites, 3 ounces lean beef patty, 1 small banana.
Calories: 428   Protein: 47 grams   Carbohydrate: 29 grams
Fat: 14 grams
P-C-F ratio: 45-26-30

Meal 2
1 cup cantaloupe cubes (eaten first), 1 cup salad topped with 6 ounces tuna, 1/4 avocado.
Calories: 359   Protein: 47 grams   Carbohydrate: 22 grams
Fat: 10 grams
P-C-F ratio: 51-24-24

Meal 3
Maxi-Burn Protein Drink (see Recipes, Chapter 17), plus 5 amino acid capsules.

Meal 4
8 cucumber slices, 8 ounces skinless chicken breast, 2 ounces raw pumpkin seeds.
Calories: 535   Protein: 63 grams   Carbohydrate: 31 grams
Fat: 17 grams
P-C-F ratio: 48-23-29

The above menus are for anyone desiring to *burn it to the max!* These menus will lower bodyfat dramatically and may be employed by competitive bodybuilders, runners, cyclists or anyone who wants to eat a low cholesterol, low fat, low carbohydrate, adequate protein, HIGH ENERGY DIET. For men to see their abdominals "clearly defined" the *Maxi-Burn* Menus are ideal.

Note: It is not suggested to go directly from a high carbohydrate diet (a diet that is based on approximately 40-70% carbohydrates), to the Maxi-Burn Meals. Most individuals find it to be a more comfortable transition into fat burning by utilizing the *Mini-Burn* Meals and the *Mega-Burn* Meals for a period of 1-12 months.

Chapter 8

Creating Your Own Meals

It is easy to design your own delicious meals by following a few simple guidelines which will insure that you consistently access fat for fuel. P-C-F balance is critical to the fat burning process. Protein must always remain adequate to facilitate fat burning while sparing lean muscle tissue. Carbohydrate should not comprise over 25% of a meal's total calories (with 20% or less being ideal) or fat burning becomes limited or is completely shut down by the release of excess insulin into the bloodstream. Fats must be high in essential fatty acids and balanced with the protein content of each meal.

All "unfriendly" fats including fried foods, margarine, roasted nuts, and high heated oils should be avoided as well as "unfriendly" carbohydrates including juices, sugar, starches, grains, cereals, all sweeteners, candy and refined foods.

In general, a typical fat burning meal could contain approximately 30-55% complete protein, 15-20% non-starchy carbohydrate and 25-55% "friendly" fats and oils. The above ratios are not absolutes, but general percentages. As calories increase or decrease according to your individual needs, the protein and fat ratios may change slightly, but carbohydrates should remain at 20%, or less, of total calories as stated earlier.

Athletes need more protein, so be aware of this fact. The strength athlete's calorie ratio may be as follows: 45% protein, 20% carbohydrate and 35% fats and oils. For attaining ultra low bodyfat (i.e. 6-8% for men and 10-12% for women), the dietary profile may look like this: 55% protein, 20% carbohydrate, 25%

fats and oils., which would be a low fat, low carbohydrate, low calorie, adequate protein diet plan.

If you have hypoglycemia, Candida or hyperglycemia then you may desire to create meals that are lower in carbohydrate or void of fruit, at least for the first 30-90 days. Limit fruit intake and increase vegetables and salads for your carbohydrate needs and please consult your physician before making any dietary changes.

Figuring dietary percentages is an easy process that only requires some simple arithmetic. Protein and carbohydrate each equal four calories per gram, while fats and oils equal nine calories per gram. To calculate your dietary percentages, simply refer to the food chart in this chapter which shows the protein, fat and carbohydrate content of individual foods. If you design a meal that is 45 grams of protein, 25 grams of carbohydrate and 20 grams of fat, your dietary percentages would be as follows:

45 x 4 = 180 calories from Protein
25 x 4 = 100 calories from Carbohydrate
20 x 9 = 180 calories from Fats and Oils
460 = total calories

Now simply divide each of the individual calorie totals by 460 to discover your protein to carbohydrate to fat percentages.

180 divided by 460 equals .39 (39%) Protein
100 divided by 460 equals .22 (22%) Carbohydrate
180 divided by 460 equals .39 (39%) Fat

From the above profile, a person who is not athletic but sedentary would need to merely lower carbohydrates slightly at this meal to correct the balance. A long distance runner could keep the ratios as they are. An athlete who is training with weights may need to slightly lower the carbohydrate percentage to 15-20%, double or triple the portions and eat four to five meals per day to keep protein levels adequate while maintaining optimum fat burning status.

You will also notice that calories are quite low on this diet, yet you will be very satisfied because you are accessing fat for fuel. This is one reason I feel *The Fat Burning Diet* needs to become universal to our planet. By utilizing fat as their primary source of energy, the human population could eat nearly half as much food and gain twice as much energy. And with world hunger, this could be one viable solution which could feed more people on much less food!

If precisely calculating meals is simply "not your bag", then you may design your own meals in a similar pattern as outlined in the *Mini-Burn, Mega-Burn* and *Maxi-Burn* plan. **Pay very close attention to the number of grams of carbohydrate you are ingesting. Keep it to approximately 1.5 grams of carbohydrate per meal for each 10 lb. of lean body weight, while also eating adequate protein to satisfy your daily needs.** For a person whose lean weight is 110 lb., they would be ingesting approximately 16.5 grams of "friendly" carbohydrates at each meal (11 x 1.5 = 16.5). With the addition of 1-3 tbs. of fresh flax oil daily and the consumption of wholesome proteins, the fats and oils equation is usually covered automatically.

From simple observation, *The Fat Burning Diet* is a low carbohydrate, low calorie, natural fat, natural protein diet. You will be eating less, burning fat, gaining strength, and discovering new energy reserves. If *fat* is not your "cup of tea" then create a low fat diet or follow the *Maxi-Burn Plan*. If you are a bodybuilder, up the protein to meet your growing needs.

If you are a runner, create smaller fat burning meals that will help you run farther and faster. While the average person will get fat fast on a diet that is higher than 25-30% carbohydrate, long distance runners and endurance athletes can often eat as much as 30-40% of their calories as "natural" carbohydrate and still burn fat effectively.[16] In fact, Dr. Barry Sears of Marblehead, Massechusettes and Dr. Phillip Maffetone of Solana Beach, California both feel that endurance athletes do very well eating a diet which is 30% protein, 40% carbohydrate and 30% fat.[17] While I feel the above dietary ratios to be slightly excessive in carbohydrate, I leave it up to my readers to determine exactly what works best for them. If you are an endurance athlete, try increasing your carbohydrate intake slightly until your performance begins to drop, then simply lower your "carbs" until performance becomes optimum. A little trial and error should produce the exact results desired.

If your busy schedule only allows you time to eat two meals per day, design larger meals with enough calories that will sustain you for six or more hours. Be creative and shape *The Fat Burning Diet* into a program that works for you. The sky truly is the limit when you allow your body to select fat as its primary source of fuel.

Fat Burning Food Chart

Abbreviation Key: Amt. = Amount; Prot.= Protein; Carb.= Carbohydrate; Cal.= calories; g.= Grams; oz. = ounce; tsp.= teaspoon; tbs.= tablespoon; C = cup.

Note: All meats listed are broiled, roasted or baked, not fried. All amounts listed are approximations.

FOOD GROUP I

Protein Foods	Amt.	Cal.	Prot./g	Carb./g	Fat /g.
Swordfish	3.75 oz.	164	27	0	5.5
Ocean Perch	4.5 oz.	128	24	0	2
Tuna (water packed)	4 oz.	120	28	0	2
Chicken Breast	3. oz.	198	29	0	7.5
Skinless Chicken Thigh	3.5 oz.	216	27	0	11
Skinless Chicken Meat	4 oz.	215	33	0	8.5
Skinless Turkey (dark)	4 oz.	210	32	0	8
Skinless Turkey (light)	4 oz.	160	34	0	1.5
Ground Turkey Patty	2.3 oz.	194	23	0	11
Beef Round Steak	7 oz.	470	52	0	27

Beef Sirloin -choice	4 oz.	320	32	0	21
Beef-T-Bone Steak	4 oz.	322	26	0	23
Beef, Lean Ground	3 oz.	240	24	0	15
Beef, Xtr Lean Ground	3.5 oz.	265	28	0	16
Deer/Venison	4 oz.	178	34	0	4
*Large Whole Egg	1 each	75	6.25	.5	5
Egg White (cooked)	1 each	16.5	3.5	.35	0
Egg Yolk (cooked)	1 each	59	2.75	.3	5
Blue Cheese	1 oz.	100	6	.5	8
Cheddar Cheese	1 oz.	114	7	.35	9
Colby Cheese	1 oz.	111	6.75	.75	9
Cottage Cheese (reg.)	4 oz.	115	14	3	5
Cottage Cheese (lowfat)	4 oz.	82	14	6	2.5
Cream Cheese	2 oz.	198	4	1.5	20
Sour Cream	2 oz.	124	4	2.5	12

*Raw eggs should be dipped in boiling water for 45-60 seconds to destroy avidin (a non-essential amino acid that interferes with biotin absorption). The best eggs to purchase are from farms that don't give their chickens drugs (growth hormone, steroids, antibiotics, etc.) and allow their chickens to move around and a "have a life".

FOOD GROUP II

Vegetables	Amt.	Cal.	Prot./g.	Carb./g	Fat/g.
Asparagus Spears (raw)	6 each	20	2	4	.2
Broccoli (raw)	4 oz.	32	3.5	6	.4
Brussels Sprouts (raw)	4 oz.	49	4	10	.3
Cabbage (raw)	4 oz.	28	1.5	6	.3
Carrots (raw)	1 each	31	.75	7	.1
Cauliflower (raw)	4 oz.	28	2.25	6	.3
Celery (raw)	4 oz.	18	1	4	.2
Collards (raw)	4 oz.	35	1.75	8	.25
Corn on Cob (boiled)	1 each	71	2.5	17	.5
Cucumber Slices	1 oz.	3	.2	.5	.3
Dandelion Greens (raw)	4 oz.	51	3	10	.8
Escarole (raw)	4. oz.	19	1.5	3.75	.2
Kale (raw)	4 oz.	57	3.75	11	.8
Kohlrabi (raw)	3.5 oz.	25	1.5	6	.1

Vegetables	Amt.	Cal.	Prot./g.	Carb./g.	Fat/g.
Iceberg Lettuce (raw)	1.5 oz.	5	.5	1	.75
Romaine Lettuce (raw)	1 oz.	3	.3	.5	.04
Butter Lettuce	1 each	45	3.75	8.5	.74
Mustard Greens (raw)	4 oz.	30	3	5.5	.2
Onions (raw)	4 oz.	43	1.5	10	.2
Parsley (chopped-raw)	1 tbs.	1.4	.1	.2	.03
Parsnips (raw-sliced)	1 tbs.	6.25	.1	1.5	.03
Green Peas (raw)	4 oz.	190	12	35	.5
Green Bell Peppers	1 oz.	7.75	.25	1.75	.05
Chili Peppers (hot-red)	1 oz.	11	.6	2.75	.06
Radishes (red-raw)	4 each	3	.1	.6	.1
Spinach (raw)	4 oz.	25	3.25	4	.4
Summer Squash (raw)	8 oz.	20	1	5.5	.1
Tomato (medium, raw)	1 each	26	1	5.75	.4

FOOD GROUP III

Fresh Fruit	Amt.	Cal.	Prot./g.	Carb./g.	Fat/g.
Apple (medium)	1 each	81	.275	21	.5
Applesauce (unswtnd.)	4 oz.	48	.2	13	.06
Apricots (pitted)	3 each	51	1.5	12	.4
Avocado (raw)	6 oz.	306	3.75	12	30
Banana (medium, raw)	4 oz.	104	1.2	26	.5
Blackberries (raw)	8 oz.	118	1.6	29	.9
Blueberries (raw)	8 oz.	127	1.52	32	.9
Red Raspberries (raw)	8 oz.	111	2	26	1.25
Strawberries (raw)	8 oz	68	1.4	16	.8
Cantaloupe (raw)	12 oz.	119	3	29	1
Grapefruit (medium	.5 each	37	.75	9	.1
Peach (medium)	1 each	37	.6	10	.1
Pear (medium)	1 each	98	.7	25	.7
Pineapple (raw)	8 oz.	111	.9	28	1
Plum (medium)	1 each	36	.5	9	.4
Prunes (dried)	4. oz	270	3	71	.6
Honeydew (raw)	1 oz.	99	1.3	26	.3
Kiwifruit (raw)	1 each	46	.75	11	.3
Mango (medium, raw)	.5 each	67	.5	18	.3
Orange (medium, raw)	1 each	62	1.25	16	.2
Watermelon (6"x 2" slc)	1 each	170	3	40	1.3

FOOD GROUP IV (A)

Nuts and Seeds	Amt.	Cal.	Prot./g.	Carb./g	Fat/g.
Almonds (raw)	4 oz.	668	23	23	60
Brazil Nuts (raw)	4 oz.	744	17	14.5	76
Cashews	1 oz.	163	4.5	9	13
Coconut (dried)	4 tbs.	129	1.5	5	13
Macadamia Nuts	1 oz.	199	2.5	4	21
Mixed Nuts (roasted)	1 oz.	168	5	7	15
Peanuts (dry roasted)	4 oz.	663	27	24	56
Pecan Halves (raw)	1 oz.	189	2.2	5	19
Pine Nuts (raw)	1 oz.	146	7	4	14
Pistachio Nuts (raw).	4 oz.	655	23	28	55
Pumpkin Seeds (raw)	1 oz.	126	5	15	5
Sesame Seeds (raw)	1 oz.	162	5	7	14
Sunflower Seeds (raw)	1 oz.	161	6.5	5	14
Walnuts (English, raw)	10 each	130	3	4	12

FOOD GROUP IV (B)

Fats and Oils	Amt.	Cal.	Prot./g.	Carb./g	Fat/g.
Butter	1 tbs.	102	.1	0	11.5
Flax Seed Oil	1 tbs.	128	0	0	14
Olive Oil	1 tbs.	119	0	0	13.5
Safflower Oil	1 tbs.	120	0	0	13.5
Canola Oil	1 tbs.	120	0	0	13.5
Wheat Germ Oil	1 tbs.	120	0	0	13.5

Dairy Products	Amt.	Cal.	Prot./g.	Carb./g	Fat/g
Whole Milk	8 oz.	138	7.5	10.5	7.5
Half and Half Cream	1 tbs.	20	.5	.5	1.75
Whipping Cream	1 tbs.	51	.3	.5	5.5
Sour Cream	1 tbs.	31	.5	.5	3
Soy Milk (plain)	8 oz.	75	6	4	4
Yogurt (nonfat, plain)	8 oz.	126	13	17	.4
Yogurt (whole, plain)	8 oz.	139	8	11	7
Cheese (Colby)	1 oz.	111	7	.75	9
Cottage Cheese (reg.)	8 oz.	233	28	6	10
Cream Cheese	1 oz.	99	2	.75	10

Starches	Amt.	Cal.	Prot./g .	Carb./g.	Fat/g.
Brown Rice (cooked)	8 oz.	251	6	52	2
Oatmeal (cooked, plain)	8 oz.	133	5.75	23	2
Corn Tortilla	1 each	67	1.75	14	.75
Pancake (wh. wheat, 5")	1 each	108	4.5	15	3.5
Bread (wh. wheat, slice)	1 each	86	3.5	16	1.5
Bagel (plain)	1 each	187	7	36	1
Corn Muffin	2 oz.	173	3.5	29	5
Waffle (plain)	1 each	218	5	26	10
Popcorn (air pop, plain)	2 oz.	216	7	44	2.5
Lasagna Pasta (cooked)	4 oz.	160	5.5	32	.75
Pasta Spirals (cooked)	4 oz.	160	5.5	32	.75
Potato (baked)	7 oz.	220	5	32	.2
Squash (winter, baked)	8 oz.	88	2	20	1.5
Sweet Potato (baked)	4 oz.	60	1	14	.1

Beans	Amt.	Cal.	Prot./g.	Carb./g.	Fat./g
Navy Beans (boiled)	8 oz.	322	20	60	1.5
Black Beans (boiled)	8 oz.	299	20	54	1
Split Peas (boiled)	8 oz.	267	19	48	1
Lima Beans (boiled)	8 oz.	261	18	47	1
Kidney Beans (boiled)	8 oz.	288	20	52	1
Tofu (plain)	3.5 oz.	75	8	2	5

Chapter 9

Cholesterol Is Your Friend, Not Your Enemy

We are at war! Pick up any newspaper, magazine or health publication and it becomes very obvious we are fighting a silent battle against CHOLESTEROL. Because cholesterol deposits itself in the arteries of heart attack victims it has been assumed that cholesterol and most fats are not healthy and should be avoided like the plague.

We have low cholesterol cookbooks, many of our packaged foods contain *no fat* and the latest buzz words are *fat-free!* With all this no-fat, low-fat, cholesterolphobia, did anyone ever stop to really take a close look at how important cholesterol is to our health and well being?

If you don't believe that diet and health are two controversial subjects, then you must be new to the field of nutrition. One study will give specific and conclusive findings that become dietary "fact". Then two years later another study will prove this fact to be completely erroneous. And I don't feel cholesterol to be any different. Look at how inconsistent the "authorities" have been on their judgment with eggs. One year they condemned eggs, the next year they are letting eggs out of prison and tell us they jumped to conclusions.

In *fact,* a recent news release stated that a panel of leading medical experts have seriously questioned the role of cholesterol in heart disease.[18] These medical authorities feel that total restriction from eating meat and dairy products is *unwarranted*. It seems that this group of doctors suddenly realized that even though specific dietary habits can alter the level of blood cholesterol, NOBODY actually knows the precise agent that causes heart disease. This panel of medical experts now believe that instead of focusing exclusively on cholesterol, a more balanced view of the connection between diet and cardiac disease should be adopted.

Cholesterol Is Vital To Your Health

Your body produces cholesterol because it is vital to your health and well being. Even if you avoid cholesterol entirely, your body will work overtime to produce your daily needs. And no matter how much cholesterol you consume daily, your body will still only absorb approximately 300-500 mg. with the remainder of your cholesterol needs being produced by your liver. In fact, through very sophisticated clinical studies it has been determined that 60-70% of **all** blood cholesterol comes from production by the liver, not from our cholesterol rich foods.[19]

Cholesterol is vitally important to every cell of the body. One of cholesterol's major roles is being the substance that your body uses in the production of steroid hormones including testosterone, estrogen, progesterone, cortisone and aldosterone.[20] Your skin contains large concentrations of cholesterol and this is where your body converts it to vitamin D in the presence of direct sunlight. Cholesterol seals off damaged tissues, arterial walls and is also needed to protect the cells of your body from being damaged by radiation, toxins and other harmful substances. Are you beginning to get the idea of just how important cholesterol is for your body?

So how did such a wonderful and vitally important substance like cholesterol get its name splattered across the front page of all the tabloids? I believe science was looking for something to blame as the cause for heart disease. Cholesterol, being found deposited in the arteries of many heart attack victims, seemed like a good place to point the finger. Cholesterol just happened to be at the scene of the crime but, in America, you are innocent until proven guilty. In my opinion, sugar, refined carbohydrates, excess carbo-hydrate consumption, processed foods, refined fats, junk food and lack of exercise are the real cause for the significant increase in heart attacks, and I believe there is a growing number of other health and fitness professionals that will agree with me on this point.

Without Cholesterol You Would Die!

All *natural* foods that contain cholesterol are loaded with leci-thin and other fatty acid mobilizing nutrients that keep cholesterol moving within the body so that it is able to accomplish its many vital functions. Without cholesterol you would die! If cholesterol is at fault and the "root cause" of heart disease, why in the world would your body be producing it in such large quantities each and every day of your life? I feel that specific nutrients are simply lacking in the diet of someone who consumes processed foods, which then causes cholesterol to behave in a "gooey" and binding manner that can eventually lead to arterial blockage, cardiovascu-lar disease, heart attack and/or stroke.

HDLs and LDLs Are Both "Good Guys"

I'm also opposed to this cholesterol labeling idea which states that HDL (high density lipoproteins) are the *good guys* and that LDL (low density lipoproteins) are the *bad guys*. This *good guy-bad guy* concept originated because your liver manufactures two carrier proteins for cholesterol. LDLs carry the cholesterol out to the tissues where it can perform its magic, while HDLs carry the cholesterol back to the liver where it is then manufactured into bile salts and prepared for excretion. LDL, being the distributor to the tissues, is often blamed for being the responsible party that places cholesterol in the arteries as the slow builder of arterial occlusions.

On the other hand HDL, by retrieving cholesterol and returning it back to the liver, which helps prevent a build-up in the arteries, has been labeled a "good guy." The truth is, HDL and LDL are absolutely necessary in the cholesterol distribution process. If labels must be applied, I see them as *both* wearing *white hats* and being *good guys* who are doing their part to maintain perfect harmony within the body.

Chapter 10

Food Combining

Food combining is a simple yet important factor that is often overlooked or left out of many diet programs and diet-related research projects. Foods are usually eaten in what ever manner and order that is customary to the individual and no care is given to eating the foods in a compatible way that could enhance both digestion and elimination.

Being controversial, the subject of food combining has been the primary fuel for many heated debates among countless nutritional authorities. One group of authorities strongly believe that eating any type of foods at a meal is natural to the human and that no care should be taken to mix and match items according to their digesting times, digestive juice needs and enzymatic capacity and specifications. The other arm of dietary "authority" absolutely feels that eating foods that digest easily together is the ideal, with one primary example being that starches should be eaten at one meal and proteins at another. Who is right? All I can say is, "No one is right or wrong on this matter."

It seems that only the affluent can afford the luxury of choosing to eat what they want, when they want it and in what manner and order they choose.

Much of the world struggles each day just to find enough to eat, much less fret over what will bring about optimum digestion. On the other hand, there is something to the idea of eating proteins at one meal and starches at another, which can be personally proven by simply trying the technique. If it works for you then do it!

Enzymes and digestion go hand in hand. A strong digestive tract will digest almost anything thrown its way, while a weakened system will sometimes sputter and balk at the simplest of foods. Most raw foods digest easier than cooked foods, which means that raw foods and cooked foods each have their own food combining and digesting rules. Fat slows digestion, making it highly beneficial as a control mechanism that facilitates the gradual release of carbohydrate into the bloodstream.

Once Starches Are Removed From One's Diet, Fat Burning Is Enhanced

The Fat Burning Diet pays close attention to simple food combining knowledge. My personal experience, along with countless numbers of my clients, has proven that proteins digest best when separated from starches. In fact, almost everything digests better when separated from starchy foods. With most starches being *cooked* (enzymatically dead) carbohydrates, possessing rapid blood sugar elevating potential, it only seems natural to severely limit or totally leave this food group out of our daily diet. And the avoidance of most cooked, starchy foods is one major point that separates *The Fat Burning* Diet from so many other diets on the market. Once starches are removed from the diet, fat burning is enhanced plus digestion and elimination are greatly improved.

It is also interesting to note that, just like starches, "sweet" foods don't combine well with proteins. Sweet foods, besides miscombining with most proteins and elevating glucose levels rapidly, also feed Candida (yeast) organisms that are living within the colon and warm, moist regions of the body. *The Fat Burning Diet* avoids starches and sweet foods and this is the true secret for this diet's great success.

Personal study, existing research and practical experience has revealed that digestion is optimum when specific food combinations are utilized while certain other food combinations are avoided. As stated earlier, a strong digestive system will attempt to digest foods in any combination and will usually accomplish this feat successfully. But to consistently maintain optimum digestion and pure elimination for one's entire lifetime, certain rules must be followed to enhance the body's food processing abilities.

The following is a list of tips to increase digestive powers of the body. And a powerful digestive system means a powerful organism.

1. **Avoid or limit starches of all kind**, including: "unripe" bananas, rice, bread, potatoes, yams, squash, cereals, grains, pasta, etc. Starchy foods do not combine well with protein or most fruits. Starches combine very well with fats and oils, sweet fruits, honey, maple syrup, and vegetables, all of which (excluding vegetables, fats and oils) will shut down fat burning in a matter of bites! Plus a properly combined starch meal is void of protein foods that should be present at each meal to feed your muscles and internal organs. A properly combined starch meal means fat storage, muscle atrophy and no fat burning activities. Bottom line: avoid or limit starches and burn fat faster. Reserve all your starchy meals to your once per week "free-for-all."

2. **Proteins, vegetables, fruit, nuts and seeds all combine very well at any given meal.** Due to the starchy nature of "unripe" bananas (which contain green on the skins, versus "ripe" bananas which are housed in skins that are **all** yellow with brown speckles) and the high carbohydrate content of dried fruits, these fruits should be avoided.

3. **Eat melons at the beginning of your meal.** If any variety of melon is consumed at a meal, eat it at the very start of your meal. Melon digests very quickly and passes on to the small intestines. Melons, when eaten with other foods, are held up in the stomach and often ferment, causing gas, bloating and stomach upset.

4. **Avoid milk.** Milk, unless fermented as yogurt, cheese or cottage cheese, is high in lactose, which is milk sugar. Many individuals are intolerant of lactose and experience cramping, gas, indigestion and sometimes even diarrhea. Fermented dairy products are usually very, very low in lactose or are completely lactose free due to the enzymatic conversion. Milk also does not combine with any other foods, so please, do yourself a favor and avoid milk.

5. **Nuts and seeds should be soaked in water for 24 hours before consuming**. Raw nuts and seeds can become heavy in the stomach, if consumed in large enough quantities, due to the presence of sprouting regulators which science has labeled as enzyme inhibitors. Raw nuts and seeds contain these enzyme inhibitors which prohibit them from germinating and hinder our digestive abilities. Water releases the enzyme inhibitors, which is nature's way of letting a new plant come to life because H_2O is the catalyst that initiates the germination process.

   Once the inhibitors are released, the seed will then be in the first stage of sprouting and may be consumed without interference to our digestive process. Twenty-four hours of soaking in pure drinking water is required for the complete release of all enzyme inhibitors present in the nut or seed.[21] Roasting nuts and seeds also releases (destroy by heat) the enzyme inhibitors. Roasted nuts and seeds are not recommended for regular consumption because heat alters and/or destroys the delicate essential fatty acids which were present in the raw state.

Chapter 11

Your Support System:
Family, Friends and the Rest of the World

"There is something in the Universe that responds to intrepid thinking."
— Ralph Waldo Trine

The strength of this unique and effective diet program resides within you. When we make changes in our lifestyle, it would be wonderful if the whole world (including family and friends) smiled upon us and supported our every effort. But that is mere fantasy, or wishful thinking, because those who are closest to us are often the least supportive of our efforts and positive changes. I am not suggesting that family and friends are never supportive, it just is rare to be praised and commended by your closest companions.

Perhaps the lack of support by family members and close friends stems from the notion that these people know you very well and simply do not wish to see you change. Jealousy, fueled by the fact that you are taking charge of your life and *they* are not, may also be a contributing factor for your most intimate acquaintances not patting you on the back.

No matter what the reason for your "social circle's" lack of support, it is vitally important that you believe in yourself and your *purpose*. Self-confident thoughts and beliefs are what cause the *Universe* to respond to our needs. Think positive thoughts that are aligned with your true purpose and the doors will open.

If you can find a purpose, a deep purpose, for utilizing *The Fat Burning Diet*, then the support will be there. The support and praise may come from the least expected areas of your life, but it will be there. Once you become successful, nearly everyone will be patting you on the back, but during the first steps of your journey, look inward for your inner strength.

For myself, *The Fat Burning Diet* came as an answer to my prayers. I was seeking the ultimate diet that could end hypoglycemia, maintain muscle mass and energize my body without fail, thus allowing me not only to live with unlimited energy but to have energy reserves to teach this diet worldwide. It takes constant, steady energy to travel, talk, lecture, workout and work 10-15 hours per day. It is imperative that I use fat for fuel, because I just can't trust those ol' carbs anymore. They always let me down faster than a leaky boat in a rainstorm.

Be open to discovering how *The Fat Burning Diet* will energize your body and act as a catalyst for making your dreams come true. The sky is the limit when you're burning fat, so get out there and go for it! With these thoughts alone, the *Universe* will respond immediately.

Chapter 12

Candida, Colon Health and Lactobacteria

Running "symptomatically" parallel to hypoglycemia is the 20th century health problem which is commonly called Candida, short for Candida albicans, which is a type of yeast that naturally resides in the colon of every healthy human.[22]

Candida organisms are thriving in the 12 foot tube that connects our small intestines to our anus. Lactobacteria also reside in a healthy colon, and are antagonist to Candida albicans. The presence of high *friendly* Lactobacteria activity in the colon helps keep Candida and other *unfriendly* bacteria in check. Both forms of bacteria must be present in a healthy colon, but the key here is to maintain the proper balance.

The healthy ratio for friendly bacteria to harmful bacteria is approximately 80% friendly to 20% unfriendly.[23] Lactobacteria are also vital to good health because they keep our bowel movements smooth, soft and healthy, plus they produce small amounts of B-12 along with an ample supply of digestive enzymes.[24]

Antibiotics and Birth Control Pills Destroy Lactobacteria

With modern day lifestyles, poor eating habits, the use of drugs **(especially antibiotics and birth control pills, both of which destroy Lactobacteria)** and worldwide air pollution, our friendly bacteria population may become diminished. In some cases, the friendly-to-unfriendly-bacteria ratios may even become reversed, indicating a serious imbalance within the intestinal tract.[25]

Once Candida and the "unfriendly guys" begin to dominate the colon, your insides start to get *ugly* (as if the inside of your colon isn't ugly enough already). With the *Candida gangs* ruling your intestinal neighborhoods, Lactobacteria simply can not flourish.

Some of the possible results of a low Lactobacteria count are: stagnation of fecal matter, gas, poor bowel movements, constipation, diarrhea, bloating, poor digestion, fatigue, dizziness, exhaustion, yeast infections, and skin rashes. With many of the above afflictions festering in your alimentary canal, poor or incomplete elimination is often the final outcome and slimy or messy bowel movements can become the norm. In time, poor elimination can create a build-up of stagnant, slimy matter in the large intestine and then you've got "trouble my friend, right here in colon city!"

A distended lower abdomen is very common to women with colon stagnation, especially after child bearing years. Sometimes the entire abdominal region is engorged (on men this is often referred to as a *pot belly* or *beer belly*) indicating that old matter has accumulated in the intestines. Both of the above examples can be easily distinguished from merely having tummy fat by simply grabbing your abdominal region with both hands. If a large handful of fat can be grabbed and the stomach muscles below are flat and tight, then you are just fat. But if very little fat can be grabbed, yet your stomach appears as if you swallowed a small watermelon, then what you could be experiencing is intestinal stagnation, Candida, gas, bloating or all of the above.

Candida and Hypoglycemia Are Identical Problems

The symptoms of Candida are almost identical to hypoglycemia, and I believe them to be one of the same afflictions. Most hypoglycemia sufferers experience gas, poor digestion, poor elimination, constipation, and a whole array of problems that almost exactly duplicate Candida symptoms. And it's no wonder; both ailments are aggravated by eating excess quantities of carbohydrates. (I have experienced both Candida and hypoglycemia simultaneously and believe them to be two different terms for the same affliction). Eliminate excess carbohydrates from your life (as *The Fat Burning Diet* suggests) and Candida and hypoglycemia will lose their life support system, which is a high level of glucose in the blood.

Colon Health

Many nutritionists blame intestinal stagnation on "mucus" and support this belief with the "mucus theory" which claims that most foods (except fruits, vegetables and sprouts) are mucus forming to one degree or another (with protein-based foods rating very high on the mucus list). The mucus theory seems logical at first glance, but once it is put to the test, it fails to produce the predicted "mucus" response. For example, cheese (according to the mucus theory) is rated high on the mucus chart, meaning that if it is consumed, this food will cause noticeable quantities of mucus to be produced by the body to protect you from the cheese. Four ounces of cheese should cause you to constantly clear your throat, spit up mucus and perhaps even have a bout of constipation from all the "mucus glue" your body will form.

High Carbohydrate Foods Are The Real Problem

And sure enough, every time you eat a pizza with lots of cheese, you do get many of the above predicted responses. Toasted cheese sandwiches too, will cause a sizable amount of mucus to suddenly appear and may even congest a few noses. But don't jump to conclusions and blame the cheese! Eat cheese alone or with low carbohydrate vegetables and where is the mucus? It never shows up! Eat zero fiber eggs (also rated high on the mucus charts) and you should be spitting up balls of mucus and be "plugged up" for a week. Right? Wrong! The mucus never appears unless high carbohydrate foods accompany the protein food that is claimed as mucus forming.

My experience with the *mucus theory* is that the consumption of sugar and excess carbohydrates of any type are the real reasons the body can't digest fat and protein foods efficiently and thus is the underlying cause of slimy bowel movements, mucus production, constipation and colon stagnation.

The Colon Can Become Plastered With Slime

During the course of our lives, most of us have had at least some exposure to antibiotics, birth control pills and less-than-optimum foods, such as desserts, ice cream, candy bars, soda pop and junk food. And the final outcome of these dietary habits is often poor digestion and elimination. Once lactobacteria activity is suppressed and a poor diet takes hold, then the colon can quickly become plastered with slime, which dehydrates over time and can block the natural flow of fecal matter.

The removal of stagnant material is sometimes necessary to create an optimum environment for Lactobacteria to thrive. Special herbal formulas taken in conjunction with a psyllium husk blend is one method for ridding the colon of old matter. The author has employed this method with great success and actually expelled many pounds of old matter using the proper herbs and psyllium powder blend. A few herbs which aid in the intestinal cleansing process are: Chickweed, Irish moss, cloves, plantain, rosemary, bayberry bark, and corn silk extract. To help remove old stagnant matter during the cleansing it is important to take a psyllium husk powder mixed with spirulina and dandelion root. Onion powder may be added to the psyllium husk formula to enhance Lactobacteria production during the cleanse.

Controlling Candida

Candida loves sugar! In fact Candida thrives on high levels of glucose in the blood. If a person ever desired to starve Candida, the first step is to cut out all excess carbohydrates in the diet. This keeps blood glucose levels in a normal range, meaning there is no "excess" to feed the Candida yeast. Consequently Candida albicans organisms die, and die fast! And, by eliminating excess carbohydrates in your diet, your body will begin to access fat for fuel. Imagine that! By cutting out all high carbohydrate foods, Candida is controlled, hypoglycemia is avoided and you begin to burn your own bodyfat as high powered energy. Nothing could be finer!

Chapter 13

Fat Burning For the Whole Family

While it is often easy for one family member to change his or her diet, expecting the rest of the family to follow suit is another matter entirely. Perhaps one of the biggest challenges, concerning diet change, is getting the kids to eat healthy foods that are low in sugar and concentrated carbohydrates.

Children, especially young children ages one to eight, can usually eat more natural carbohydrates than adults and "get away with it", meaning that a child is active enough to burn most of the excess carbohydrates in their diet. An optimum diet for children limits or restricts all refined sugars and refined carbohydrates and leans heavily toward a balanced diet of complete proteins, non-starchy vegetables, fruits, nuts, seeds and occasional whole grains and starchy vegetables.

But how in the heck can you get your children to eat correctly, especially in this day and age? Just do your best. The sooner you introduce your children to "whole foods" the better. Restricting all sugar, sweets, candies and excess carbohydrates can be a difficult task. Peer pressure combined with TV ads, and an early developed "sweet tooth" will almost always keep your child's hand in the cookie jar.

Raising A Healthy Child Is Fun!

Our son Angelo was born at home, in an underwater birth, and has been raised with love, attention and plenty of organically grown whole foods. Being breast fed from day one and receiving nothing but raw fruit and breast milk for his first year, our son got off to a very healthy start in life. White sugar has graced his lips less than a handful of times during his five years of existence, while whole foods have been his mainstay. All this special care and dietary focus has produced a beautiful child who is calm, considerate and free of illness. I am not relating this story of my son Angelo to merely brag about how wonderful he is. It is being shared with you to point out that it is possible to raise a "natural child", even in "junk food" replete America.

Carbohydrates Are Everywhere!

From soda pop to pizza, refined carbohydrate temptations are everywhere. Right in your own home is the first place to begin weeding out the "junk." Go through your cabinets and perform a serious refined carbohydrate cleanse. Get rid of all the ooey, gooey products that are going to give you and your family an insulin rush. Next replace all the "junk" with "real" foods. Begin developing meals that are centered around proteins and vegetables. Stop serving potatoes, pasta and macaroni and cheese as main courses and focus on salads, steamed vegetables and choice protein selections.

You Deserve The Absolute Best!

Buy organically grown foods to insure that what you serve your family is not chemically poisoned and deficient in nutrients. And this goes for meats too! Buy hormone free meats that come from animals which are fed natural foods and are raised under humane and healthy conditions. Ask the Manager of your local supermarket to carry the above types of clean, pure foods.

For desserts, utilize many of the low carbohydrate treats you'll find in the Recipe Chapter. Choose vegetables, nuts, seeds and fruit as your child's natural carbohydrate sources. Try to limit "starchy" foods (bread, pasta, rice, potatoes, etc.) as much as possible, but there is no need to go overboard. Some whole grains are just fine for "active" children and will do no harm (unless they are allergic to the food itself, such as wheat which is a highly allergenic grain for many humans).

Make Dietary Transitioning Fun

Do your best to raise your children on whole, unrefined foods, but don't force the action. Let it "flow", especially if radical dietary changes are necessary. Forcing your children to change against their will can often create a resentment toward wholesome food and perhaps end in complete rebellion. Keep it "light" and make dietary transitioning a fun and memorable experience for the whole family.

Chapter 14

Exercises That Burn Fat

"Exercise addicting is often the result of food (carbohydrate) addiction. By breaking your addiction to carbohydrates, you automatically end your addiction to exercise."

If you are exercising regularly and not restricting carbohydrates in your present diet, then there is a strong possibility you could be addicted to your daily workout. Why? Because high carbohydrate diets often force a person to engage in glucose burning activities to by-pass the fat storing cycle (caused by excess glucose in the bloodstream). That plate of pasta will soon be stored as fat unless you can "run it off." Your activities, coupled with insulin's action, burn excess sugar in your blood which stops the fat storing process before it can begin.

There are many problems with eating a high carbohydrate diet and combining this with intense daily exercise.

1. Burning excess glucose in the bloodstream along with glycogen stores in the muscles can take one or more hours of very intense aerobic activity. Due to the presence of high concentrations of insulin in the bloodstream, little if any fat is mobilized and burned as fuel.

2. Exercise becomes addictive as you must rely upon it as an antidote to your carbohydrate addiction. Carbohydrate addiction stimulates exercise addiction which is employed to control weight gain caused by the eating of excess carbohydrates.

Stop The Insanity! Eat Fewer Carbohydrates!

On a high carbohydrate diet you "must " workout or else get fat. And don't think thin individuals get away with eating excess carbohydrates either. There are many "skinny" people who have very high bodyfat levels (I know, because I was one of them). Excess carbohydrates just love to become "fat" (triglycerides) and then seek every opportunity to "hang out " with you.

Exercise can be employed to control a high carbohydrate diet. But what happens if you miss a workout or, heaven forbid, you become injured and can't workout at all for 4-6 weeks? Blimp City right? On a high carbohydrate diet the answer is a strong "Yes!" On *The Fat Burning Diet* the answer is a clear cut NO! Without excess carbohydrates in your life, lay-offs are no threat to your bodyfat percentages. By following *The Fat Burning Diet* principles you will break all carbohydrate addictions which automatically breaks all exercise addictions.

The Best Exercises for Burning Fat

Long, slow to medium speed motions are optimum fat burning activities. This means a 30-50 minute workout is ideal and should be performed 3-5 days per week. The exercises one chooses to perform are entirely up to the individual. The bottom line for burning fat while following *The Fat Burning Diet* principles is to burn fat calories, so simply get into motion! Go for regular walks, ride your bike, buy a skateboard, strap on your rollerblades, or go surfing. Just go do it and you'll burn more fat!

When your body is accessing fat for fuel, any motion (except short bursts of speed, such as sprinting) will increase the fat burning process. Covert Bailey, in his book, *Fit or Fat*, used the analogy of fat being a log, and carbohydrate is the kindling. Trickle in small amounts of carbohydrate (kindling to start the fat burning process), and the fat (log) will burn long and steady. Dump in too much carbohydrate and you get a flash fire that flares quickly and then burns out.

Calculating Your Fat Burning Target Heart Rate

To consistently burn fat while exercising, simply maintain a "target" heart rate that is approximately 70% of your maximum heart rate for your age and physical condition. Calculating your "target" heart rate is very simple. Subtract your age from 220 and multiply the remainder by 70% and the final figure will be your "fat burning target zone", which is the number of heart beats you need to maintain per minute of exercising. You then try to remain within a 5% range, either way, of your "target" heart rate throughout your entire aerobic workout.

Take your pulse at 3-5 minute intervals during intense exercise. Your pulse may be monitored by placing your index and middle finger on the underside of your wrist or at either side of your neck, 1/2 inch to the right or left of your windpipe. Count the number of beats for 10 seconds and multiply by 6 to calculate your heart rate. This method requires a little practice to perfect, but after 3-4 tries most individuals develop the skills that are necessary to accurately monitor their heart rate.

If taking your pulse is difficult or inconvenient, you may desire to utilize an electronic heart rate monitor which may be purchased from your local sporting goods store. Prices may range from $50-150 dollars per monitor, with the higher priced, chest-strap models usually possessing the highest degree of accuracy.

Note: Unless your are employing an electronic heart rate monitor, you will need to stop exercising for a few brief moments to take your pulse. This will not adversely affect your training intensity or exercise productivity. Once you have attained an accurate pulse reading, simply resume exercising at the necessary pace that places you within your "target zone."

My Personal Fat Burning Exercise Routine

I presently exercise 3 days per week for approximately 50-60 minutes per session. A typical workout might be 15 minutes on the stationery bike (or a 1.5-2 mile run), followed by 35-45 minutes of progressive resistance weight training. Coupling my exercise routine with *The Fat Burning Diet,* I stay toned, trim and happy! And by choosing to burn fat for fuel I have plenty of energy for oodles of other activities. On some days I'll go for a brisk walk, or I'll take the family to the beach for a day of fun in the sun. Other days I'll throw the Frisbee in the park, go bike riding, mow the lawn or do what ever else I choose. When you're burning fat, activities become easy and down right exciting. Ain't life grand!

Chapter 15

Fat Burning For Bodybuilders and Athletes

"Behind all success, there is a dream. The greater the dream, the greater the success."

The ultimate dream of the bodybuilder is to gain muscle while losing fat, which makes *The Fat Burning Diet* ideal for anyone that lifts weights. Powerlifters and bodybuilders across the nation simply love the effects this eating program has on their physiques. Burning away fat while gaining muscle size and strength is often expressed as the most thrilling by-product of following my program.

As a former gym owner, long time personal trainer and now fitness consultant, I have had the opportunity to work "one-on-one" with hundreds of individuals who all dream of fitness success. I've seen countless young, aspiring bodybuilders never attain their goals and dreams simply because they refused to change their diet and lower their bodyfat. It seems that everyone wanted to "get big" and forgot that "big" means "muscle enlargement", not fat expansion.

To get the "look" of a bodybuilder, an individual must become defined, meaning they must lower their bodyfat to approximately 6-8% for men and 10-12% for women. Once the bodyfat has been lowered, the muscles of the bodybuilder are then visible and the body becomes a work of art. *The Fat Burning Diet* is the ideal way of eating to ensure low bodyfat and maximum muscle size.

You'll Reach Your Dreams and Beyond!

In my opinion, there is no other diet on the market which can produce such dramatic results in such a short period of time. If you have been training hard for years and have yet to attain the "bodybuilding look" that you desire, then give this diet a try and I guarantee you'll reach your dreams and beyond.

Lost 80 lb. of Fat Without Losing Any Strength!

A "drug-free" competitive powerlifter phoned me recently to profess his delight with *The Fat Burning Diet*. His former weight of 275 lb. had been reduced by 80 lb. which allowed him to compete in the 198 lb. class. His sheer delight came from the fact that he had not lost any strength. In other words, he was still squatting and dead lifting over 600 lb. on each lift, yet he was 80 lb. lighter! In fact, he felt so strong and had chiseled so much fat away, he was even considering becoming a competitive bodybuilder.

If you are an endurance athlete, *The Fat Burning Diet* will help you tap into your fat reserves faster and more consistently than ever before, thus giving you an edge on those "long hauls." You can stop chewing those "endurance candy bars", start eating real foods and begin using your own fat for fuel. Remember, at 10% bodyfat your body will contain approximately 10-30 times as much energy as fat than it does as carbohydrate, so why not burn your fat and save your carbs?

Thirty minutes before going on a long run or bike ride, try eating a small fat burning meal of approximately 12 grams of protein, 10 grams of carbohydrate and 6 grams of "friendly" fats or oils. Personal experience has shown that the above meal ratios will spark the hormonal response desired to activate fat mobilization within the body. Insulin will only trickle into the bloodstream while glucagon will pour forth to initiate the fat burning process.

Your small fat burning meal may be a protein drink which contains the following ingredients: 6 ounces pure water, 1/2 ounce egg white or milk and egg white protein powder, 10-12 strawberries (or any other type and amount of fruit that contains approximately 10 grams of carbohydrate), 1/2 tablespoon flax seed oil. Place all ingredients in an electric blender and mix for 30 seconds, then drink. This same drink may be duplicated and consumed after your long run or bike ride to replenish the system and continue the fat burning process. Two other simple fat burning meals, that you could consume before a workout, would be a 4 ounce dish of whole milk cottage cheese and 4 grapes or two eggs and 1/4 of an apple.

Chapter 16

Flaxing Your Muscles

Do you crave foods high in fat? Do you suffer from dry skin that needs oiling on a daily basis? Have you ever followed a low fat diet? Do you make protein drinks with a non-fat protein powder?

If you answered yes to any of the above questions, then you need to know about a great new food product called flax seed oil. Flax oil is actually a highly nutritious oil that has been around for centuries. When this special oil is combined with a high quality protein, the synergistic effect could be equated to MUSCLE DYNAMITE!

Many hard training athletes follow a diet that is high in complex carbohydrates, moderate in protein and low in fats. Egg whites, non-fat milk products and non-fat protein powders are the rage because we are taught to believe that low fat intake will translate to low body fat. But a diet too low in fat can be detrimental to our health. Constipation, eczema-like skin eruptions, kidney problems, susceptibility to infections, sterility in males, retardation of growth, and overall weakness are just a few of the problems that can stem from a diet that is too low in fats (the essential fatty acids).

In his highly informative book, *Fats and Oils,* author Udo Erasmus explains, from a scientific point of view, that a diet high in protein but low in fat is as degenerative as is a diet high in fat and low in protein. In other words, if animals were given diets deficient in protein and or the "essential" fatty acids, then death came quickly.

In 1902, a study showed that a high carbohydrate, low protein diet resulted in fat deposition. A high carbohydrate, high protein diet also was found to cause an increase in fatty deposits. But when "good" fats were added into the same diets, less fatty deposition occured and better food utilization and energy production took place.[26] To put it to you straight, essential fatty acids help us to burn fat, which is contrary to the average American's way of thinking.

A "friendly" fat contains BOTH of the essential fatty acids, linoleic acid (LA) and linolenic acid (LNA). This precious partnership of essential fatty acids can only be found in a few choice foods (usually nuts and seeds) which is one reason *The Fat Burning Diet* includes liberal portions of both nuts and seeds (unlike so many other diets that are very low in fat and limited in essential fats and oils). And because the essential fatty acids are extremely perishable, the food sources we choose to obtain them from must be FRESH, because heat (cooking), light (storage) and oxygen (open containers) destroy their beneficial properties.

One of the best "friendly fats" to choose while following *The Fat Burning Diet* is fresh, cold pressed (very few bottled oils are actually pressed without heat) flax seed oil, because it contains both essential fatty acids and is especially high (57-60%) in linolenic acid (LNA).[27] Flax oil is best used when mixed with a high sulfur source of protein such as, cottage cheese, eggs or a non-carbohydrate egg white or milk and egg white protein powder.

Protein Drinks Taste Delicious When Mixed With Fresh Flax Seed Oil

In my personal experience with flax oil, I prefer to use one tablespoon on a fresh vegetable salad, and top this with a squeeze of fresh lemon or lime. Many of my famous protein drink recipes include a high quality egg white or milk and egg white protein mixed with fresh flax oil. To the best of my knowledge, I am the first fitness professional to ever advocate flax oil in protein drinks.

Most typical protein drinks are made with non-fat ingredients (including the protein powder) which renders the combination unsuitable for muscular growth. Add in 1 tablespoon fresh flax oil to each protein drink and not only will your muscles be happier but your overall health will soar to new heights!

Fat Cravings Ended!

There will be no more "low fat blues" when flax oil is used daily in your diet. Many years ago I craved fatty foods of all types. (I believe, at that time, I was essential fatty acid deficient). After I began including 2-3 tablespoons of fresh flax oil into my daily diet, all my unhealthy fat cravings ended. For the first time in my life I was fat satisfied and felt completely balanced.

Flax seed oil is not a heavy fat either. It will keep you feeling light and actually enhance your daily workouts because both LA and LNA substantially shorten the time required for the recovery of fatigued muscles after exercise. This is accomplished by the fact that LA and LNA are facilitators for the conversion of lactic acid to water and carbon dioxide.[28] Hello better shape, good-by soreness!

Where can you obtain fresh flax seed oil? Many natural food stores now carry flax oil in the refrigerated department (flax oil should be refrigerated when possible, and especially after opening). Flax oil is highly perishable (like all oils) and must be fresh pressed (all good flax oil is dated to ensure freshness) and stored in black plastic or dark amber glass containers. *The Fat Burning Diet* utilizes flax seed oil extensively because of its high nutritional value.

Chapter 17

Delicious Fat Burning Recipes

Nothing is more delightful than creating delicious meals from "scratch" utilizing whole foods that form a combination of nutrients that, once eaten, will allow your body to access fat for fuel. It's like having your cake and eating it too! (Sorry, no cake on this diet. Instead we have "Banana Dream Pies!"). And it is even more exciting to know that all the fat burning meals you prepare are going to energize yourself and anyone else that should partake of these delicacies.

Being prepared is important if you are going to have fun in the kitchen. Nothing is more frustrating than to get halfway into a recipe and realize one or two of the necessary ingredients are not on hand. The following is a partial list of items that you will need to create many of the fat burning recipes in this chapter:

- one 8 inch Teflon skillet
- one 12 inch Teflon skillet
- one sauce pan
- one colander (for rinsing)
- one set of measuring spoons
- one measuring cup, one or two cup capacity
- one sharp knife
- one cutting board
- spices including: basil, cayenne pepper, garlic powder, onion powder, parsley flakes, chili powder.
- a variety of natural liquid flavorings including: banana, almond, strawberry, cherry, and vanilla.

- a blender
- a mixing bowl
- several large spoons
- a mixer with rotating blades.
- Nutrasweet brand sweetener (for desserts)
- a natural barbecue sauce (no sugar, no salt)
- mustard (no salt)

It has been a blast creating, and then enjoying, all the delicious recipes for this book. It gives me even greater pleasure to now be able to share them with you. Giving is the true joy of life!

Each recipe is presented to you under a heading that suggests the meal that it represents, but please feel free to indulge in any of the meals or recipes whenever your tastes and schedule dictate. Omelets for dinner or a protein drink for lunch is quite common to my personal menu plan. To achieve maximum fat burning, each recipe may be combined with other foods to form a complete meal that contains ample protein, "friendly fats" and is limited in carbohydrate. All protein drink recipes are already balanced and catagorized for your convenience.

Main dishes may be served with a salad and a small piece of low carboydrate fruit to form the proper fat burning balance. Recipes that suggest serving sizes are for a 170 lb. active male who lifts weights. Adjust the portions to suite your own calorie needs.

The Recipes Are Fun and Easy To Prepare!

Do not imagine that these special Fat Burning recipes can only be mastered by a trained chef or the "woman" of the household. Guys and unskilled "kitchenites" will have absolutely no problem whipping together these simple, yet delicious recipes.

Feel free to truly enjoy yourself as you dance through the kitchen, tossing salads, buzzing blenders and creating "triglycerides torching" masterpieces. And once you fully adapt to the basics of *The Fat Burning Diet*, you will be able to create your own special dishes. Please feel free to share any of your fat burning recipes with me. I love to discover new creations and master-pieces from fellow fat burners around the world. Send all mail correspondence to:

Jay Robb Enterprises • Fat Burning Recipes • Box 711533
Santee, CA 92072-1533

And now, for the moment you have all been waiting for, hhheeeeres the recipes...

Egg Dishes

Cheese Omelet (Mini-Burn) Serves 1
Calories: 376   Protein: 27 grams   Carbohydrate: 2 grams
Fat: 29 grams

2 large eggs
2 oz. cheese, sliced (no salt if possible)

1. Preheat an 8 inch Teflon skillet over medium-low heat.
2. Crack both eggs into a bowl and whip with a fork until blended smooth.
3. Pour the eggs into the heated Teflon pan then tilt the pan until the eggs cover the pan evenly.
4. As soon as the eggs are solid, place the cheese slices on 1/2 of the eggs and fold the other half of the eggs on top of this.
5. Slide the half circle omelet onto a plate and serve with fresh salsa or your favorite pasta sauce. For a special treat, sprinkle with 1 teaspoon lecithin granules.

Turkey Breast Omelet (Mega-Burn) Serves 1
Calories: 503   Protein: 45 grams   Carbohydrate: 2 grams
Fat: 34 grams

2 large eggs (cracked in a bowl and whipped with a fork)
3 oz. turkey breast (cooked and sliced)
1 green onion (chopped)
1 tbs. olive oil
1 oz. cheese (grated)

1. In an 8 in. Teflon pan, sauté the olive oil, green onion and turkey breast on low-medium heat for 2-3 minutes until the onion is just barely crisp.
2. Pour the eggs into the Teflon skillet, tilt until the eggs cover the entire pan surface and cook until the eggs just become solid.
3. Sprinkle the omelet with the grated cheese, then fold in half and slide onto a plate. Top with salsa or thin slices of fresh tomato.

Spinach Omelet (Mini-Burn) Serves 1
Calories: 523   Protein: 28 grams   Carbohydrate: 8 grams
Fat: 42 grams

2 large eggs (cracked in a bowl and whipped)
3 large spinach leaves (washed and chopped)
2 oz. cheese (grated)
1/2 small white onion (chopped fine)
1 tbs. olive oil
1 clove of fresh garlic (chopped)

1. Place the olive oil, onion and garlic in an 8 in. Teflon skillet and sauté until the onion begin to brown. 2. Pour the eggs into the pan and tilt the pan to spread them evenly.
3. Place the spinach on top of the eggs and cover the pan.
4. As soon as the eggs are just solid, sprinkle the omelet with

grated cheese and fold in half. Then slide it from the pan onto a plate and enjoy!

Hot Diggidy Dogger (my son Angelo's favorite) (Mega-Burn)
Serves 1

2 large eggs (cracked into a bowl, taking care not to break the yolks).
2 Shelton's brand turkey or chicken hot dogs (sliced into pieces while frozen).

1. Place the sliced hot dogs in a low-medium heated Teflon skillet and cook until thawed and warm.
2. Gently slide the eggs onto the hot dogs and tilt the pan until the egg whites cover all the hot dog slices.
3. Cover and cook until the egg whites are solid and the yolks are still runny (sunny side up).
4. Carefully loosen the eggs from the pan with a Teflon spatula and slide onto a plate. Top with salsa, avocado slices and chopped green onion if desired.

Tune A Omelet Supreme (Maxi-Burn) *Serves 1*
Calories: 287   Protein: 41 grams   Carbohydrate: 3 grams
Fat: 11 grams

4 egg whites, 2 yolks (beaten together in a bowl)
1/2 can (3 1/4) oz. water packed tuna (drained and chopped)
1 tsp. lecithin granules
1 green onion (chopped)
1 clove garlic (chopped)
1/4 cup pure water

1. Sauté the onions and garlic in water in an 8 inch Teflon skillet heated low-medium.

2. Add the beaten eggs and sprinkle with lecithin granules and the chopped tuna.

3. Cover and cook until the eggs are just firm, then fold over and slide the omelet onto a plate and serve.

Turkey Time and Sunshine (mega-burn) Serves 1
Calories: 497   Protein: 42 grams   Carbohydrate: 2 grams
Fat: 34 grams

4 large eggs
2 oz. turkey (cooked and sliced thin)
1 tbs. olive oil

1. Place olive oil and turkey in a Teflon skillet and sauté for a few minutes.
2. Crack the eggs into the pan and take care not to break the yolks.
3. Cover the pan and cook until the whites are solid and the yolks are runny (sunny side up).

Super Salads

Veritable Veggie Salads will be the main constituent of your lunch and dinner meals. Utilize a wide variety of fresh vegetables when creating your own fat burning salads. The combinations are almost infinite. Here are some of my favorite blends...

Cabbage Patch Power (maxi-burn) Serves 1
Calories: 187   Protein: 36 grams   Carbohydrate: 6 grams
Fat: 2 grams

1/4 head green cabbage (sliced very thin)

3 red radishes (sliced thin)
2 green onions (chopped)
4 oz. turkey breast (cooked and diced)

1. Place the sliced cabbage on a plate and spread evenly.
2. Add the radishes and green onions in a colorful manner.
3. Top with the diced turkey and cover with 1 tbs. of your favorite salad dressing.

Taco Salad (mega-burn) Serves 1
Calories: 442   Protein: 36 grams   Carbohydrate: 17 grams
Fat: 26 grams

1/4 head lettuce (chopped or sliced thin)
1/8 head green cabbage (sliced thin)
1/2 tomato (diced)
10 cilantro leaves (pluck leaves from the stems)
1/4 medium size ripe avocado (peeled and sliced thin)
4 oz. extra lean (8-12% fat) ground beef (browned in skillet)
1/2 yellow onions (chopped)
1 tsp. chili powder

1. Brown the ground beef with the onion and chili powder.
2. Spread the lettuce and cabbage evenly on a large plate.
3. Cover lettuce and cabbage with the ground beef mixture
4. Add the chopped tomato and cilantro leaves.
5. Top with fresh salsa and the avocado slices.
(This is one of my favorite dinners!)

Tuna Salad Supreme (maxi-burn) serves 1-2
Calories: 354   Protein: 44 grams   Carbohydrate: 4 grams
Fat: 17 grams

1 - 6 1/4 oz. can of water packed, no salt tuna (drained)
1 green onion (chopped)
2 red radishes (sliced)
1 stalk celery (chopped)
1 tbs. mustard (no salt)
1 tbs. olive oil or flax oil
1/8 tsp. cayenne pepper

Place tuna in a medium size bowl and cover with onion, radishes, celery, oil and cayenne pepper. Mix together well and serve with a sprig of parsley.

Dynamo-Dinner Ideas

Mega-Burn Meat Loaf (mega-burn) *serves 6*
(per serving) Calories: 451   Protein: 47 g.   Carbohydrate: 5 g.
Fat: 26 g.
2 lb. extra lean ground beef
2 tbs. chili powder
4 egg whites, 2 yolks
2 cloves of garlic (diced)
1 large onion (chopped)
1 tbs. parsley flakes
4 tbs. tomato paste

1. Preheat oven to 375 degrees.
2. Place ingredients, except tomato paste, in a large bowl and mix thoroughly.
3. Place meat loaf in an oil baking dish and cover with the tomato paste.
4. Bake 50-60 minutes.

Green Bean-Burner (mega-burn) *serves 2*
(per serving) Calories: 507   Protein: 65 g.   Carbohydrate: 16 g.
Fat: 21 g.
3 cups fresh green beans (end clipped and cut in half)
1/4 cup raw almonds (chopped in a blender)
12 oz. turkey breast (cooked and chopped)
2 oz. raw, unsalted cheese (grated)

1. Steam green beans for 10-15 minutes until tender.
2. Place cooked beans, evenly divided on two plates.
3. Cover with almonds and cheese, then toss lightly and serve.

Chicken Breast Bonanza (maxi-burn) *serves 6*
(per serving) Calories: 277   Protein: 47 g.   Carbohydrate: 2 g.
Fat: 8 g.
2 lb. boneless, skinless chicken breasts
1 tbs. parsley flakes
1 clove garlic (chopped)
1 tbs. olive oil
1 medium onion (sliced thin)
1/2 lemon (sliced thin, no seeds)

1. Preheat oven to 375 degrees.
2. Place chicken breasts in a deep baking dish.
3. Cover chicken with olive oil, parsley flakes, garlic, onion slices.
4. Top with lemon slices, cover dish with aluminum foil and bake
for 30-40 minutes.

Navel Orange Roughy (maxi-burn) *serves 6* (per serving)
Calories: 260   Protein: 38 g.   Carbohydrate: 1.5 g.   Fat: 13 g.

2 lb. orange roughy (thawed if you purchase your fish frozen)
1 tsp. garlic powder
1/2 navel orange (sliced)

1 tbs. parsley flakes
1 tbs. olive oil

1. Place orange slices in a broiling pan lined with aluminum foil.
2. Place the orange roughly on top of orange slices.
3. Cover the fish with olive oil and sprinkle with parsley and garlic.
4. Broil for 12-15 minutes, taking care not to overcook.

Delicious Protein Drinks

All protein drinks must be made with an egg white protein
powder or a milk and egg white protein powder that DOES NOT
contain added carbohydrates. Purchase a basic formula protein
powder and read the ingredients disclosure very carefully. DO
NOT purchase protein powders that contain soy, or isolated soy
protein (these proteins are inferior and often cause gas and/or
indigestion to their users).

To mix the protein drinks, place all ingredients in a blender and
blend until creamy smooth (about 45 seconds). All drinks are one
serving unless otherwise stated. Add ice or freeze the fruit if a
frosty cold drink is desired.

NOTE: *Raw eggs should be dipped in boiling water for 45-60
seconds to destroy avidin, a non-essential amino acid that interferes with biotin absorption). The best eggs to purchase are from
farms that don't give their chickens "drugs" (growth hormone,
steroids, antibiotics, etc.) and allow their chickens to move around
and a "have a life".*

Protein Power! *(maxi-burn)*
8 oz. pure water
1 cup ripe strawberries (frozen OK)
.5 tbs. flax seed oil
1.5 oz. protein powder
Calories: 266   Protein: 37 g.   Carbohydrate: 14 g.   Fat: 7 g.
P-C-F ratio: 55-20-25

Tropical Treasure *(mega-burn)*
6 oz. pure water
1/2 small papaya
1 egg
1 tsp. lecithin granules or liquid
1.5 oz. protein powder
1/2 tsp. coconut extract
Calories: 326   Protein: 43 g   Carbohydrate: 16 g   Fat: 10 g.
P-C-F ratio: 53-19-28

Inner-G Supreme *(mega-burn)*
3 oz. pure water
1 orange (juiced)
1 tbs. flax seed oil
1.5 oz. protein powder
1 egg
1/2 tsp. pineapple extract
Calories: 412   Protein: 43 g.   Carbohydrate: 15 g.   Fat: 20 g.
P-C-F ratio: 42-15-43

Strawberry Sunrise *(mega-burn)*
6 oz. pure water
1 cup strawberries
2 eggs

1 oz. protein
Calories: 301   Protein: 37 g.   Carbohydrate: 15 g.   Fat: 14 g.
P-C-F ratio: 50-20-30

Fat Burner Supreme (mega-burn)
6 oz. pure water
1 peach (pitted)
1 tbs. flax oil
1.5 oz. protein
1/2 cup strawberries
Calories: 342   Protein: 37 g.   Carbohydrate: 17 g.   Fat: 14 G.
P-C-F ratio: 43-19-38

Vanilla I Scream Delight! (mini-burn)
4 oz. fresh cream
1 egg
2 oz. pure water
1 ripe banana (frozen)
1.5 oz. protein
1 tsp. pure vanilla
Calories: 745   Protein: 46 g.   Carbohydrate: 37 g.   Fat: 48 g.
P-C-F ratio: 24-20-56

Bod-E-Builder (mega-burn)
8 oz. pure water
3 eggs
2 oz. protein
1 banana (frozen)
1 tsp. lecithin (granules or liquid)
Calories: 567   Protein: 68 g.   Carbohydrate: 28 g.   Fat: 20 g.
P-C-F ratio: 48-20-32

The Famous "Banana Delight" (maxi-burn)
(a Jay's Gym classic!)
8 oz. pure water
1 ripe banana (frozen)
1 tbs. flax seed oil
2 oz. protein powder
1 egg
Calories: 506   Protein: 55 g.   Carbohydrate: 27 g.   Fat: 20 g.
P-C-F ratio: 44-21-35

Maxi-Burn Delight! (maxi-burn)
8 oz. pure water
1 tsp. lecithin (granules or liquid)
1/4 cup frozen blueberries
2 oz. protein powder
1/2 tbs. flax oil
1/2 small banana
Calories: 400   Protein: 49 g.   Carbohydrate: 18 g.   Fat: 15 g.
P-C-F ratio: 49-18-33

Bodybuilding Mass Builder (mega-burn)
10 oz. pure water
6 eggs
1/2 cup frozen strawberries
1 ripe banana
2 oz. protein powder
1 tbs. flax oil
Calories: 930   Protein: 87 g.   Carbohydrate: 44 g.   Fat: 45 g.
P-C-F ratio: 38-19-44

Peaches and Cream (mini-burn)
6 oz. pure water
3 oz. fresh cream
1 egg

1 ripe peach (pitted)
2 oz. protein powder
Calories: 643   Protein: 57 g.   Carbohydrate: 22 g.   Fat: 37 g.
P-F-C ratio: 35-14-51

Specialty Recipes

Homemade Sauerkraut
2 heads of green cabbage
1 earthenware crock

1. Cut the cabbage into very thin strips and place in crock until you have a layer about 3 inches deep.
2. Then tamp this down very well with a clean 2 x 4 piece of wood, then add the rest of the cabbage doing the same until the cabbage is really pressed in tight. There must be no air present between the cabbage pieces!
3. Cover this with a clean piece of cheese cloth and a thick paper plate. On top of this place a 10 lb. weight or a one gallon jug of water to give the mixture constant pressure.
4. Place the crock somewhere warm (75 degrees Fahrenheit) and leave undisturbed for 7-10 days.
5. When the sauerkraut is ready, divide evenly (including the juice) and refrigerate in glass jars for storage.

This recipe is even easier if made in a Japanese pickle press that may usually be purchased from your local health food store.

Homemade Whipped Butter
8 oz. raw cream or heavy cream
1. Place cream in a mixing bowl and whip with electric beaters until it turns to whipped cream.
2. Continue whipping until very stiff and is of whipped butter consistency.
3. Cover and refrigerate.

Fresh Salsa (maxi-burn)
3 tbs. flax seed oil
3 tomatoes (chopped fine)
4 sprigs of fresh cilantro
1/2 medium onion (chopped)
1 green onion
1 small jalapeno pepper (chopped)
1/2 cup tomato sauce (sugar and salt free)

1. Place all ingredients in a large bowl and mix together with a large spoon.
2. If you like your salsa hot, then use 2 jalapeno peppers.

Delicious Fat Burning Desserts
(these are fun foods for special occasions and are not to be used on a regular basis)

"Real" Whipped Cream
8 oz. raw cream or whipping cream
1/2 tsp. vanilla
1 tbs. Nutrasweet (optional)

1. Place all ingredients in a mixing bowl and whip with electric beaters until the cream becomes stiff. Do not over whip or this will turn to butter.

Banana Dream Pie (mini-burn) serves 8
Calories: (per serving) 221   Protein: 17 g.   Carbohydrate: 9 g.
Fat: 14 g.
P-C-F ratio: 30-17-54
Filling:
1 cup water
1 package unflavored gelatin (Knox is a good brand)

2 tbs. Nutrasweet brand sweetener
1 1/2 ripe bananas
3 oz. egg white protein powder
4 eggs (dipped in boiling water for 1 minute)
1/2 pint fresh cream
1 tbs. flax seed oil
1 tsp. vanilla extract

Crust:
1 cup raw almonds (or English walnuts)

Utensils Needed:
1 blender
1 small sauce pan
1 measuring cup
1 set of measuring spoons

Approximate Preparing Time:
15 minutes

1. Place 1/4 cup of room temperature water in a saucepan and sprinkle with gelatin. Let stand one minute at room temperature, then stir until dissolved using low heat. Set this aside.
2. In a blender, add one cup raw almonds and blend on low until chopped fine. Lightly coat a 9 inch pie pan with butter and pour the chopped almonds in the middle, then spread them evenly to make a crust. Set this aside.
3. Using the same blender add the: 4 eggs; remaining 3/4 cup water; bananas; Nutrasweet; protein powder; cream; vanilla; flax seed oil; and the 1/4 cup of dissolved gelatin (that you set aside).
4. Blend for 45-60 seconds until smooth and pour contents into the almond crust pie pan.
5. Cover with clear plastic wrap and place in the refrigerator for 3 hours until gelatin is completely set.

This truly is a Dream Pie that will not give you a sugar rush. For variety, substitute 8 oz. of cream cheese for the cream to make a Banana Cheese Cake. For a holiday treat cover the pie, after it has set, with fresh whipped cream and sprinkle with a few tablespoons of chopped almonds.

Cottage Cheese Supreme (mega-burn) *serves 1*
6 oz. lowfat cottage cheese
1/2 cup strawberries (sliced)
6 shelled walnuts halves
1 tbs. fresh whipped cream (optional)

1. Place cottage cheese in a bowl.
2. Cover with strawberries, nuts and top with whipped cream.
Calories: 277   Protein: 26 g.   Carbohydrate: 19 g.   Fat: 44 g.
P-C-F ratio: 37-19-44

Cinnamon Apple Delight (mini-burn) *serves 1*
6 oz. lo-fat cottage cheese
1/2 apple (peeled, cored and diced)
6 shelled walnuts halves
1 tsp. flax seed oil
Ground cinnamon
1 tbs. whipped cream (optional)

1. Place cottage cheese in a bowl.
2. Cover with apple, flax oil and walnuts.
3. Top with whipped cream and sprinkle with cinnamon to taste.
Calories: 339   Protein: 26 g.   Carbohydrate: 19 g.   Fat: 18 g.
P-F-C ratio: 30-22-48

Super Salad Dressings

Mixing Instructions: Place all listed ingredients for each recipe into a blender and mix for 30-45 seconds on medium. Store the dressings in the refrigerator.

Italiano Supreme
1/2 cup olive oil
1/2 cup pure water
1 clove garlic (diced)
1/2 lemon (juiced)

Flax Attack!
1/2 cup flax seed oil
1/2 cup pure water
1 clove garlic (diced)
1/2 lime (juiced)
3 oz. cream cheese

Creamy Supreamy
1/4 cup olive oil
1/4 cup flax oil
1/4 cup water
2 egg yolks
1/2 orange (juiced)
2 oz. cream cheese

Cheesie Italian
1/2 cup olive oil
2 cloves garlic
3 tbs. apple cider vinegar
5 oz. cream cheese
add water to regulate consistency

Hot to Trot
1/2 cup cottage cheese
1/2 cup flax oil
1 egg yolk
1/2 cup pure water
1/8 tsp. cayenne pepper
1 clove garlic (diced)

Zesty Tomato
1/2 cup olice oil
1/4 cup pure water
1 ripe tomato (peeled)
1 green onion (diced)
1 clove garlic (diced)

Chapter 18

Mini-Cleanses for Maximum Health

Fast One Day Per Month

It is important for adults to abstain occasionally from eating, thus allowing the body to rest. Your digestive organs are working constantly and deserve to take a break. For the purpose of complete rest, I recommend that everyone take one day per month and fast, meaning that you do not consume anything for a 24 hour period, except water. This means no juice, no fruit, no coffee and no tea. Just pure spring or distilled water as thirst dictates and rest as much as possible.

An accomplished and efficient fat burner will have no problems during this one day absence from food. For the fat burning individual, it will be a day of level energy, very little hunger and a feeling of peace as the internal organs rest and recuperate. Try to sip water throughout the day and you may drink anywhere from two quarts to one gallon, depending on your size and the climate.

Eat a Protein Only Meal Several Times Weekly

While small amounts of carbohydrates are needed to avoid ketosis, utilizing a protein only meal every few days does not usually plunge a person into ketosis and can be very invigorating, cleansing and Candida suppressing. Choose one meal, and then only consume protein foods that contain almost no carbohydrate (examples: chicken, fish, turkey, eggs, beef, cheese, etc.). Eat enough at your protein only meal to become satisfied and then for your next meal simply resume back to *The Fat Burning Diet Plan.*

Chapter 19

Nutritional Supplements

Nutritional supplements are just that, nutrients that supplement a person's diet. Supplements do not replace foods, they enhance foods, or sometimes correct nutritional deficiencies

There are literally thousands of nutritional supplements on the market. Vitamins, minerals, herbs, protein powders, carbohydrate drinks and homeopathic remedies are just a few examples of common nutritional supplements.

There Are No "Magic Pills" That Burn Fat

There are no known supplements that actually burn fat, so don't expect to purchase a bottle of pills that will magically dissolve your fat. Fat burning is a metabolic process that is triggered by the amount and type of foods we eat combined with the amount and type of physical activities we are engaged in daily. Nutritional supplements do enhance the fat burning process by supporting the system's need for specific nutrients that mobilize and manipulate fat into a ready to burn medium. High quality protein powders are also useful to the fat burning process because they insure that fat, not muscle tissue, is being burned. Protein powders must not contain carbohydrates and must be blended according to the recipes listed in Chapter 17.

For general health insurance, it is advisable to make a comprehensive multiple vitamin and mineral pack a part of your daily life. It is best to consume these packets with the evening meal to insure maximum absorption and utilization of the nutrients.[29] Please consult your health care provider and your local natural food store for a vitamin and mineral blend that is suitable for your personal needs.

In conjunction to a multiple vitamin and mineral formula, there are specific nutrients that support the system as it burns fat. The following nutrients may be consumed two times daily, one dose with each meal:

Choline.............................500 mg. - Prevents fats from accumulating in the liver and facilitates the movements of fats into the cells. Choline also improves memory, is essential to healthy myelin sheaths of the nerves and helps to prevent gallstones.

Inositol.............................500 mg. - Aids in the metabolism of fats and helps reduce blood cholesterol.

L-Methionine..................250 mg. - Aids in cleansing the liver and keeping the system clean during the fat burning process.

Lecithin.............................100 mg. - Same as Choline and Inositol.

Betaine HC1.....................100 mg. - Aids in digestion, especially of fats and proteins.

Vitamin C.........................500 mg. - Maintains collagen, helps wounds heal and gives strength to the entire system.

Chromium Picolinate......200 mcg. - Restores the efficiency of insulin by affecting GTF (glucose tolerance factor).

L-Carnitine.......................250 mg. - Necessary for the transport of fatty acids. Also helps to lower triglycerides and raise HDL levels of the blood.

Egg white protein...........1 oz. - A premium source of protein that is important for growth and repair of muscle tissue, internal organs, hair, nails, etc. (may be used as a meal itself by mixing according to the protein drink recipes found in Chapter 17)

Flax seed oil.....................1 tbs. - Contains both essential fatty acids and is especially high in linolenic acid (57%)

While it is not specifically a supplement, I recognize the importance of consuming plenty of pure water each day. Fat burning is a process that requires water. If we restrict our water intake then the fat burning process is impaired.

Pure water..................1 qt. to 1 gal. daily - Essential to the fat burning process as well as all bodily functions. Also prevents constipation, which is often caused by colon dehydration due to low water intake.

Occasionally you may face moments of stress, or an energy slump, especially as you transit into becoming an efficient fat burner. For those times or during any time of physical or mental stress try taking the following:

Desiccated liver tablets, 1500 mg. - High in all the B-vitamins and contains an anti-fatigue factor that has never been isolated. Take 5-10 tablets or more during times of stress, or during an energy slump. Bodybuilder and athletes often consume 15-30 tablets per day to boost recovery from exercise.

Chapter 20

Fat Burning Questions and Answers

Q. How much weight will I lose on your diet, and at what rate will I lose it?

A. I do not refer to the results attained on this diet as "weight loss", simply because the main purpose of the diet is to burn fat as fuel, thus creating "fat loss", not weight loss. Weight loss could be attributed to water loss, lean muscle loss and/or fat loss. By restricting carbohydrates and targeting your fat cells as a source of sustainable energy, *The Fat Burning Diet* stimulates "fat loss" and absolutely minimizes lean muscle loss, which is just the effect you need for maintaining your precious strength and energy levels. How much "fat" you can expect to lose and how fast you will lose it really depends upon several factors: a) the amount and type of carbohydrate you intake, b) your present level of fitness, c) the amount of calories you expend each day, d) the amount of calories you intake each day. My clients usually average 2 lb. of fat loss per week, if they are not physically fit when they begin the diet. For my clients that are already in very good condition, fat loss may be as high as 3 lb. per week initially.

Q. Is The Fat Burning Diet nutritionally balanced?

A. The Fat Burning Diet is very nutritionally balanced. By including whole foods, ample protein, wholesome fats, raw vegetables, raw fruits, raw nuts and raw seeds, this diet excels in nutritional content. Also, by avoiding poor food combinations (the diet excludes starchy foods which do not combine with protein foods) you will not only be eating a highly nutritious diet, but your digestion will be greatly improved, thus insuring that the nutrients are readily available for absorption and utilization within the body.

Q. Why do you keep stressing the importance of not eating too many carbohydrates each day? Will a cup of rice or two pieces of toast really be a problem?

A. While eating starchy foods such as pasta, bread, rice or cereal is far from the ideal, as long as the amount of carbohydrate is within the given limits at each meal you will still burn fat. Many people don't realize that a cup of cooked rice is approximately 38 grams of carbohydrate or that a plate of pasta could be 80-100 grams of carbohydrate. One bagel "carbs in" at a whopping 30 grams and one small pancake is 23 grams of carbohydrate. Besides being easy to blast out of your carbohydrate range, grains and starches are common foods that many individuals are allergic and/or addicted to, with wheat topping the list of problem foods. Do yourself a favor and skip the starches for the first two months of the diet and then reintroduce them gradually if you feel they still need to be a part of your life. It is also best to rotate all starchy foods, never consuming any one given type more frequently than every 5 days. By rotating your starchy carbohydrates, it will keep you from developing an allergic reaction and/or addiction to those foods.

Q. How can I be sure I'm burning fat while following your diet?

A. It's very simple. Accurately measure your bodyfat before you begin the diet and then test it again every 30 days, noting the decrease in bodyfat percentages. Have your local fitness club or medical professional test your bodyfat accurately. If you need information on in home bodyfat testing devices, please call *1-800-To-Burn-Fat.(1-800-862-8763)*

Q. I'm a bodybuilder and I want to adapt The Fat Burning Diet to my training program. Will I be able to gain muscle and lose fat at the same time? Also, what about competing? Can I lower my bodyfat to 4-5% using your low carbohydrate principles.

A. *The Fat Burning Diet* is a bodybuilder's dream come true. For muscle size and low bodyfat, just stick to the mega-burn and maxi-burn menus. For competition, utilize the maxi-burn menus only. Many bodybuilders who have followed this diet plan were thrilled to finally find a diet that gives then the "look" they have always desired.

Countless bodybuilders have become discouraged with their training progress, basically because they never achieved low enough bodyfat levels to have "cuts", which is what makes a person look like a bodybuilder. As for gaining mass, please be patient on my fat burning diet. THIS DIET DOES NOT BULK-UP A BODYBUILDER by making them fat. The weight you gain on this diet will be lean muscle mass. Patience must be exercised here also because the average amount of muscle that a drug-free bodybuilder can gain is only about one half ounce per day, which translates to approximately one pound per month totaling to 12 pounds per year.[30]

Q. I have been diagnosed as having hypoglycemia and am presently eating 6 small meals per day, consisting mostly of complex carbohydrates and low fat proteins. The only problem is that I never feel mentally stable and always crave sweets and sugary baked goods. And once I indulge in the "forbidden fruit" I become a basket case, feeling weak, shaky and down right mentally confused. Will burning fat change all this for me. I'm desperate!

A. I have personally experienced the diet you described above, which supposedly "controls" hypoglycemia, and all it did was keep me in a state of total mental and physical instability. Eating starchy complex carbohydrate foods to control a blood sugar disorder is the exact opposite approach needed for ending this problem. Switch to *The Fat Burning Diet* principles and eat only four meals per day as described. This will take you off the carbohydrate roller coaster ride that is making you a "basket case." Relief should come on the first day of the diet and get better as you practice the principles throughout your life. You should also discuss *The Fat Burning Diet* with your doctor before making any changes.

Q. Whenever I try to change my diet I get a lot of criticism from my family and my friends at work. When I make a change everyone seems to suddenly become an expert on what is best for me. I then become confused with all the advice, stop making the positive changes and revert back to my old eating habits. How does a person avoid all the criticism and negative attitudes that seems to surround a person who is in the midst of "positive" changes?

A. The best approach for avoiding criticism while making any changes in your life is to discuss your changes with ABSOLUTELY NO ONE! Don't talk about it; DO IT! Then, after 2-3 months, try discussing your changes and experiences with someone close to you. If they freak out or get heavy on you with guilt trips, fear tactics or are not supportive of your changes, drop the discussion with them immediately. Tell them you do not need their negative attitude or fears and let them be. Your changes are for yourself and no one else. What you do is your own private matter and no one else's business unless you allow it to become their business. If, on the other hand, you discuss your changes with a friend and they are excited and supportive, then keep talking to them! Find your positive supporters and spend time with them. You may find yourself with a whole new set of friends, which is exactly what happened in my life.

Many people will experience fear as they watch YOU take charge of your life and they may talk negatively about you and the changes you are making. They will try to scare you with cholesterol fear, fat fear, starvation fear, going against the grain fear, and more. And as your bodyfat levels plunge to normal or an athletic low level, many people may even try to scare you into thinking you are "wasting away!" Well fear not for, "there is nothing to fear but fear itself."

Fear is an interesting phenomenon. It doesn't really exist and is actually created in the mind of an individual. Most fears come to a person when their blood sugar levels are low and the brain is starved for glucose (actually fear **and** confusion can exist in this state of being). A "fat burner" never has this typical "fear" problem because blood sugar levels are stabilized as fat is being burned for most energy needs.

Q. I have two children ages seven and nine. They both cringe at the thought of eating "natural" foods. Can they follow The Fat Burning Diet Plan and how can I get them to stick with it?

A. Children ages 1-16 usually do best on a modified version of the Fat Burning Diet. Some starches may be allowed but use only whole food starches such as oatmeal, potatoes, yams, squash and brown rice. Try to eliminate all refined carbohydrates such as white bread, sugar, pizza, white pasta, enriched macaroni noodles, white rice, etc. Serve natural, hormone free meats, eggs and cheese, along with plenty of salads, steamed vegetables, nuts, seeds and fruit. Use starchy foods only as a final filler if your child requests them.

Many parents tell me that their children refuse to eat "wholesome" foods. I always tell them that their children are not really hungry. Have them miss a meal and give them no "junky snacks"; then watch them "belly up" to the dinner table begging for your "wholesome" foods. If a child is not hungry at a meal for "real" foods, then he or she should never be forced to eat. Usually a loss of appetite for a child means that they ate sugary or high carbohydrate snacks within 1-3 hours before the meal. Take away the "junk" and limit snacks to only sliced vegetables or fresh fruit and your child should suddenly develop a new zest for "natural" foods.

Chapter 21

In Summary

The body's fuel of choice is fat, not carbohydrate. The source of fat your body will select is either dietary fat or bodyfat. Consuming excess carbohydrates stops your body from selecting fat as its primary energy source. *The Fat Burning Diet* allows your body to access its own fat for fuel by restricting most carbohydrates while eating ample protein and healthy sources of fat.

Starches, which are concentrated carbohydrates, are the main food group that Americans consume in excess. *The Fat Burning Diet* eliminates or greatly restricts all starchy foods including bread, rice, all grains, cereals, pasta, potatoes, yams and pasta. *The Fat Burning Diet* also eliminates all simple sugars including juice, sugar, sweets, all sweeteners, dried fruits, candy, ice cream, etc. Vegetables, nuts, seeds and fruit are consumed in amounts that encourage the body to burn fat for its energy source.

By controlling the amount and type of carbohydrates ingested, the body begins to select fat as fuel on a consistent basis. It takes approximately 30-120 days for the human system to create the enzymatic network required to burn fat efficiently. During this transition time the body will occasionally experience energy slumps as it switches from glucose to fat. Once the system is efficient at burning fat, the sky is the limit and energy seems to never run out. Fat derived energy does not cause energy ups and downs, nor does it make the brain "fuzzy" between meals, as carbohydrates often do.

Hypoglycemia, diabetes Type II, carbohydrate addiction, Candida and certain food allergies are all carbohydrate-based, blood sugar disorders. *The Fat Burning Diet,* by limiting carbohydrates, helps to stabilize blood sugar levels for life, thus helping to prevent any of the above disorders from developing.

The Fat Burning Diet is far more than just a weight loss program. It is a way of life that helps put you in the driver's seat! Once you gain control of your thoughts, moods and momentary reactions by stabilizing blood sugar levels, then life becomes a calm and peaceful journey devoid of many unnecessary "ups and downs".

Unlike other weight loss programs, *The Fat Burning Diet* promotes maximum fat loss while offering unlimited energy to almost everyone who utilizes this eating plan. If weight loss is your reason for utilizing *The Fat Burning Diet,* then fat loss expectations might range from 1-2 lb. per week as a conservative average. Remember though, we target fat for fuel, so weight loss is almost all fat and very little muscle.

An individual may design *The Fat Burning Diet* so that it suits their personal tastes and needs. *The Fat Burning Diet* can be low or high in fat depending on the individual's needs, likes and dislikes. If someone is concerned about cholesterol, then the diet can be designed to be low in cholesterol. If someone is allergic to dairy products, then these may be eliminated and substituted with another source of protein. The possibilities are infinite for making this diet work for you as long as you consume only 15-20% of your total calories as carbohydrate with calorie intake being adjusted to meet your physical size and daily energy needs.

When designing your own fat burning meals, try to stick to the basics and keep it simple.

1. Keep each meal's carbohydrate percentage around 15-20% of total calories. Large salads and low carbohydrate fruit will offer you plenty of high quality carbohydrates.

2. Use plenty of variety when selecting your foods.

3. Eat 3-5 fat burning meals each day and focus on maintaining a proper balance for all your meals. If your carbohydrate consumption ever exceeds 25% of your total calories, then you will begin to seriously limit or completely inhibit your fat burning potential. If you consume refined carbohydrates, simple sugars or too much fruit, your body will be stimulated to release insulin to control the sugar rush and all fat burning will come to an immediate halt.

4. If you desire to lower your bodyfat beyond the normal range for your particular age group (10-16% for men and 12-18% for women), then simply lower your calories slightly by cutting back on a few of the fatty foods you are consuming. Select lower fat meats, skip the cheese and eat mostly from the maxi-burn menus. The above dietary suggestions will work very well for an athlete, bodybuilder or dancer who wishes to lower his or her bodyfat to a level that will enhance their performance. It is best not to lower your bodyfat levels beyond 6% for males or 10% for females, except for very short periods of time.

Chapter 22

In Closing
A Personal Testimonial

The Fat Burning Diet is more than a weight loss book. This project required over 16 years to complete and I'm continually learning new secrets that will help us all burn fat more efficiently. This diet truly is a gift from God which I am sharing with the world. That was my promise.

Eyesight Returned To Normal

We all have various needs and reasons for utilizing *The Fat Burning Diet*. By adhering to all the principles of this diet program I have corrected many health problems and recharged my entire system with a source of energy that never lets me down. At one time in my life, I needed to wear eyeglasses, and my right eye was almost considered legally blind (i.e. 20/200 vision). I now possess very close to 20/20 vision in BOTH eyes and I attribute this primarily to the fact that *The Fat Burning Diet* avoids salt and starchy foods including all grains. If these two foods ever creep back into my diet, then my vision gradually becomes impaired. It is my dream that this diet will have the same effect on others as it has on myself in this area. (I can't promise that everyone will be able to throw away their eyeglasses, but it is a prayer of mine).

During the 16 years that were necessary to develop this unique eating plan, not only did I read, study and research this project perpetually, but I also personally experienced almost every diet imaginable. By actually experiencing a wide variety of diets I was given hands-on knowledge that could not be found in any textbook. And I left "no stones unturned". A small listing (including comments) of the many diets that I experienced include:

1. One year on a 100% raw food diet of only organic fruits and vegetables (Not enough protein, too many carbohydrates, no fat burning).

2. Seven years of strict vegetarianism, with eggs and dairy included occasionally (Not enough protein unless too many starches were consumed, which in turn caused me to become rather corpulent).

3. One year of Veganism which is a vegetarian diet that contains no dairy, eggs or animal flesh (absolutely too low in vital protein and offers no fat burning activity).

4. Five years of eating 90-95% of my foods raw. (This style of eating was wonderful except that it did not contain enough protein nor could it allow me to access fat because it was too high in carbohydrates).

5. The Beverly Hills Diet (too much fruit, which completely stops all fat burning).

6. The Atkin's Diet (This diet is excellent except that too many "unfriendly" fats are allowed, making it unsuitable for athletes or anyone desiring to increase their physical performance and lower their bodyfat to an athletic level. Dr. Atkins has truly done his homework and spent many, many years working with thousands of patients. My hat goes off to this fat burning pioneer!).

7. A Typical American Diet, which consisted of a wide variety of all food types including but not limited to: refined foods, sugar, processed meats, salt, sugary soft drinks, and many whole foods (This was the worst diet offering no fat burning activity, no blood sugar stability, frequent colds, poor eyesight, tonsil infections, gas, constipation, etc., etc.).

8. Macrobiotics (Salty, cooked, dead, starchy and lifeless. Not enough protein and absolutely no fat burning activity).

9. High complex carbohydrate, low fat, low protein (This style of eating stopped fat from burning, caused Candida problems to reoccur, blurred my eyesight, gave me gas, congested my nose and sinus cavity, and caused my blood sugar levels to become very unstable and unpredictable).

In my honest opinion, *The Fat Burning Diet* outperforms every diet and eating plan that you find listed above. Your entire life will change when you begin to burn fat as your primary source of fuel. Your strength will increase, your thoughts will be clear, your bodyfat will drop and remain low, and you will never seem to run out of energy!

This book is my gift to you and it is my hope and prayer that *The Fat Burning Diet* will open new doors in your life, thus allowing your dreams to become reality. This diet and this book are two of my dreams come true.

May God bless you with energy, health and prosperity...

References

[1]G. S. Ellis, Ph.D., *Control of Food to Make Energy*, March, 1991.

[2]John Kirschmann, *Nutrition Almanac*, p.p. 144, McGraw Hill, 1979.

[3]Robert Forman, Ph.D., *How To Control Your Allergies*, p.p. 186, Larchmont Books, 1977

[4]R. C. Atkins, MD., *Dr. Atkins' New Diet Revolution*, p.p. 109, M. Evans and Co., 1992

[5]R.A Passwater, Ph.D., *The Longevity Factor, Chromium Picolinate*, p.p. 42-43, Keats Publishing, 1993.

[6]G. S. Ellis, Ph.D., *Control of Food to Make Energy*, March, 1991.

[7]Dr. B. Sears, *Diet, Endocrinology, and Fat Loss: Why You're Still Fat*, Eicotec Foods, 1993

[8]Atkins, R.C., MD., *Dr. Atkins' New Diet Revolution*, p.p. 55, M. Evans and Co., 1992.

[9]Sears, Dr. B., *The Mythology of High Carbohydrate Diets*, p.p. 12-13, Let's Play Magazine, Oct. 1991

[10]Atkins, R.C., MD., *Dr. Atkins' New Diet Revolution*, p.p. 51, M. Evans and Co., 1992

[11]Cahill, G. and Aoki, T.T. *Medical Times* 98 (1970).

[12]C. Igram, Dr., *Eat Right or Die Young*, p.p. 68-69, Literary Visions Inc., 1989

[13]South, J., M.A., *Optimal Nutrition Review*, Vol. 1, No. 1, July 1989.

[14]Colgan, Dr. M., *Optimum Sports Nutrition*, p.p. 146-151, Advanced Research Press, 1993.

[15]Santillo, H., B.S., M.H., *Food Enzymes, The Missing Link To Radiant Health*, p.p.2, Hohm Press, 1987.

[16]Sears, Dr. B., *The Mythology of: High Carbohydrate Diets*, p.p.12-13, Let's Play Magazine, 1991.

[17]Maffetone, Dr. P., *Eat Fat and Get Fast!*, PR NUTRITION, 1993.

[18]Yessis, M., Ph.D., *Performance Shorts*, p.p. 35, Muscle and Fitness, Nov. 1993

[19]South, J., M.A., *Optimal Nutrition Review*, p.p. 1, Vol. 1, No. 1, July 1989.

[20]Ibid.

[21]Howell, Dr. E., *Enzyme Nutrition,* p.p.119-120, Avery Publishing Group, 1985.

[22]Crook, W.G., MD., *The Yeast Connection*, p.p. 2-3, Professional Books, 1991.

[23]Jensen, B., DC., *Tissue Cleansing Through Bowel Management*, p.p. 74-75, Jensen, 1981.

[24]Gray, R., *The Colon Health Handbook*, p.p. 17, Rockridge Publishing Co., 1983.

[25]Jensen, B., DC., *Tissue Cleansing Through Bowel Management*, p.p. 74-75, Jensen, 1981.

[26]Erasmus, U., *Fats and Oils*, p.p. 270, Alive Books, 1986.

[27]Johnston, I. and J., *Flaxseed (linseed) Oil and the Power of Omega-3*, p.p.23, Keats Publishing, 1990.

[28]Erasmus, U., *Healing Fats...Killing Fats*, Erasmus, 1990.

[29]Mindell, E., *Vitamin Bible*, p.p. 22-23, Warner Books, 1991.

[30]Colgan, Dr. M., *Optimum Sports Nutrition*, p.p. 148-149, Advanced Research Press, 1993.

About The Author

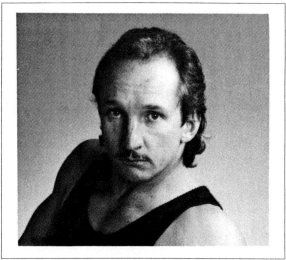

Photo by Jamal Dean

Jay Robb was born June 15, 1953. He is President of Jay Robb Enterprises, the former owner of Jay's Gym, and long time personal trainer/fitness consultant. Jay is also a feature columnist, fitness advisor and contributing editor for various prominent health and fitness magazines.

Mr. Robb is a fat burning specialist who has spent his last 16 years researching and developing fast and effective methods for clients and individuals to dramatically lower their bodyfat levels. Jay's company produce their own line of nutritional supplements and carry a full assortment of fitness products and equipment to help individuals achieve their best.

Jay, his lovely wife Rosemary and their son Angelo live in the San Diego area. He encourages everyone interested in transforming their life, through the power of fat burning, to contact him. He is available for One-On-One consultations as well as seminars. If you would like to sponsor a Fat Burning Seminar for your family, group, business or organization, or desire a personal consultation for yourself, please contact:

Jay Robb Enterprises • Box 711533 • Santee, CA 92072-1533
1-800-To-Burn-Fat (1-800-862-8763)
619/562-3787 (in the San Diego area)